The present manuscript is based on the discoveries of Prof. Dr. Enderlein. He developed a procedure for the investigation of native blood using dark field microscopy. This has been systematically reworked here and amplified in the light of the authors' personal experience extending over many years.

Introduction
into
Darkfield Diagnostics

The investigation of native blood
as developed by Prof. Dr. Günther Enderlein.

by Cornelia Schwerdtle and Franz Arnoul

Nachdruck 2022
2. Auflage 2006

Printed in Germany
Gesamtherstellung: Druckerei Adam Prettenhofer, 27324 Eystrup
ISBN 978-3-925524-47-9

Structure of Contents

Introduction

The use of dark field microscopy in the investigation of native blood was developed by the zoologist and bacteriologist Prof. Dr. Günther Enderlein (1872-1968). This particular deployment of microscopy makes it possible to observe the micro-organisms which inhabit the blood of living beings and which Enderlein discovered and described. The presence of microbes in the blood was confirmed years later by other researchers who, however, ignored Enderlein's pre-existing nomenclature (v.Brehmer, 1947; Villequez, 1956). In spite of Enderlein's discoveries having been confirmed, conventional medicine failed to give credence to the procedure which he had developed for dark field blood investigation. It was with Prof. Dr. Virchow that the saying originated: "The blood is sterile", and this is still standard teaching at universities now, as it was then. However, one look into the dark field microscope should be all that is required to convince the sceptic that the opposite is in fact the case.

Dark field blood investigation is an indispensable part of Enderlein's treatment, since this method makes it possible not only to arrive at a diagnosis but also to monitor the subsequent treatment. It is a procedure which yields precise information regarding the nature of the blood, in particular the state of the leucocytes, the erythrocytes, the plasma and the microbes contained in them. Combined with other investigative methods, it normally enables a diagnosis to be made. Furthermore, changes in the blood count which are the precursors of disease may thus be identified at an early stage, enabling appropriate treatment to be provided and making dark field microscopy a superb tool for the examination of native blood and the establishment of a precise and early diagnosis.

We can only hope that in future the potential of dark field microscopy as a basis for diagnosis will be increasingly exploited, so that patients will benefit accordingly.

1. Enderlein's Discoveries

In 1916 Günther Enderlein was doing research into the causative agent of typhus when, using dark field microscopy, he noticed tiny living organisms in the blood which were combining with more highly organised bacteria. Initially the Berlin bacteriologist could find no explanation for this observation. On searching the literature he came across the work carried out by Antoine Béchamp (1883), which had lain forgotten for years. Béchamp postulated that all animal and plant cells contained granules (granulations moléculaires) which remained alive whilst the cells were dying. Not only this, but under certain conditions bacteria were capable of changing and appearing in different forms. Thus viruses, bacteria and fungi were nothing more than different developmental stages of a particular microbial species. This so-called Pleomorphism is the polar opposite of Monomorphism, which constitutes the currently accepted teaching and practice in Biology and Medicine. Those who represented the monomorphic view, chiefly Pasteur, assumed that bacteria and other micro-organisms were incapable of manifesting in more than one form. Thus microbes were classified into various orders, families, genera and species, and each infectious illness was attributed to its own specific causative agent.

Pasteur enjoyed the greater prominence and his discoveries prevailed; Pleomorphism lay forgotten until Dunbar (1907) and Enderlein engaged in a further dispute on the subject. Enderlein discovered that all micro-organisms possess one developmental cycle, commencing with the primitive phases, moving on to the bacterial phases, then culminating in the fungal phases (see Chapter 2). Occupying the lowest position on this cycle (cyclode) we find the protite, an immobile vegetable protein colloid, and at the highest point, a fungus. Between these two poles of the cyclode innumerable growth forms are to be found, among them the various bacterial phases. In his Cyclogeny of Bacteria, which appeared in 1925, Enderlein describes the developmental cycles of numerous bacterial species and establishes a systematic structure. In later publications he gave particular attention to the cyclode of Mucor racemosus Fresen, a type of mould.

Of major significance was the proof that bacteria possess a nucleus (= mych) and are capable of reproduction in both sexual and non-sexual ways. In the twenties representatives of orthodox bacteriology contested these discoveries of Enderlein's; however they were later confirmed by observations carried out by phase-contrast and electron microscopy.

Furthermore, Enderlein refuted Prof. Virchow's dogma that "the blood is sterile". He found that a symbiont of vegetable origin is always present in mammalian blood. Enderlein called this micro-organism the endobiont or proto-symbiont, its culmination being the fungus Mucor racemosus Fresen. The bacterial equivalent is Leptotrichia buccalis. In healthy blood only primitive stages of Mucor racemosus are normally found. These colonise the blood plasma and blood cells, and all the body fluids and tissues. They have a highly significant regulatory function, with particular regard to defence and blood viscosity. The endobiont has a vital role to play in blood clotting in the form of thrombocytes (see Chapter 2).

Apart from the endobiont a further micro-organism of vegetable origin occurs in the human body. This symbiont culminates in the form of Aspergillus niger van Thieghem, whose bacterial equivalent is the tuberculosis bacillus (Mycobacterium tuberculosis, synonym Sklerothrix tuberculosis). The primitive stages of Aspergillus niger have a significant regulatory role in calcium metabolism and the citric acid cycle. Thus upward development within the Aspergillus cyclode will generally result in diseases of the skeletal system or in cancers (Arnoul, 1992).

Enderlein postulated that an infestation by developmental forms of Aspergillus niger was basic to the evolution of the vertebrates. As proof of this hypothesis he cites the most primitive vertebrate form, the lancelet (Amphioxus lanceolatus). Surviving only as a fossil, this had not developed a bony skeleton. In the course of the lancelet's phylogenetic evolution a symbiosis probably developed between the vertebrates and the primitive stages of Aspergillus niger. The latter were responsible for the calcification of the skeleton and the development of the spinal column. Thus the genesis of the bacterial form of Aspergillus niger is closely bound up with the genesis of the whole order of vertebrates, since numerous cold-blooded animals (such as turtles) are host to the tubercle bacillus and a differentiation has appeared in several species (e.g. Mycobacterium tuberculosis, Mycobacterium phlei).

Parallel to this there exists a close association between the development of the mammals and the genesis of the endobiont, which enabled the coagulation of the blood (Chapters 2 & 3).

Both symbionts are transmitted diaplacentally. They have a definite mutual relationship and can complement or replace each other.

2. Transformational Potential of Micro-organisms

In the previous chapter brief reference was made to the developmental cycles (cyclodes) of micro-organisms, as described by Enderlein. The most primitive developmental stage of each microbe is the *protite*, an immobile plant protein colloid with a diameter of approximately 0.01 µ. Enderlein described the protite as the primal manifestation or basic building block of life.

Depending on their environment, protein colloids can aggregate in various forms:

- The filum results from a one-dimensional linear arrangement of protites. Owing to its small diameter of 0.01 µ, just like the protite, this tiny "thread" is not visible under the dark field microscope.
- A two- or three-dimensional arrangement of protites results in the so-called *symprotite*, a primitive granule with a diameter of up to 1 µ.
- Another of the primitive stages is the *chondrite*, shaped like a dumb-bell and consisting of one or two symprotites and a filum. The chondrite stage is characterised by its continual alternation between filum and symprotite.
- A further form is the *spermite*, which consists of a small symprotite head with a filum and a flagellum. In 1917 d'Herelles described the spermite as a bacteriophage, without reference to Enderlein's nomenclature. The accepted thinking was that bacteria could be annihilated by these bacteriophages; however, this was refuted by Enderlein. In his view this "devouring of bacteria" was actually sexual reproduction of bacteria, in which the spermites were copulating with the primitive nuclei of the bacteria (= mych), thereby dismantling the latter into non-pathogenic stages.

By means of upward development within the cyclode the symprotites can evolve into the various bacterial stages (see Figs. 1 & 2). Enderlein designated this upward development as *probaenogeny*, or cyclogenetic ascent. During this process the symprotite accumulates a deposit of numerous protites on its surface, which serve as a food reserve. This reserve accumulation gradually increases through the addition of further protites until the point at which a spherical cell, which Enderlein called a *mychite*, emerges from it. The original symprotite now becomes the primitive nucleus (= mych) and the deposit of protites (protein colloids) becomes the cytoplasm. It is now possible for the nucleus to be surrounded by a deposit of lipoids and nucleic acid derivatives. Enderlein designated this sheath of reserve materials the *trophosome*, or *trophosomelle*; the ensemble of nucleus and sheath he called the *trophomych*.

Among bacteria, the mychite is the basic morphological unit. As development takes place, this primary form may evolve into either thecites or bacteria (Fig.1):

(a) Enlargement of the nucleus (mych) of the mychite results in a spherical cell with a polyvalent nucleus, the *cystite*. Eventually the nucleus divides, and the cystite becomes a *thecite*, a spherical cell with two or more nuclei.
(b) Following division of the nucleus and subsequent extension of the cell, the mychite develops into a twin bacillus, the *dimychite*. As development proceeds, the next stage is a quadruple bacillus, the *didimychite*, and so on. Enderlein called this alternation between single sphere and twin bacillus (rod-shaped) the *basite stage*, and the alternation between twin and quadruple bacillus the *phytite stage*. The alternation between sixteenfold and thirty-twofold bacilli he called the *ascite stage* (Fig.3). The longer forms, resembling mycelia, are growth-forms of the *mycascite stage*. In the stages named above, the primal nuclei are *catatactic*, i.e. in linear arrangement. Bacteria whose nuclei are arranged three-dimensionally were collectively designated by Enderlein as *synascites*.

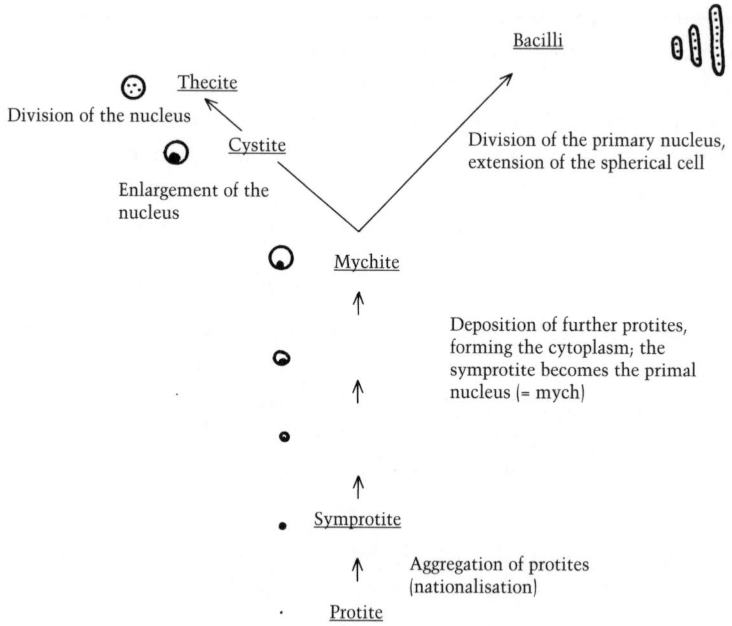

Fig.1: Development from protite to bacillus, modelled on Leptotrichia buccalis.

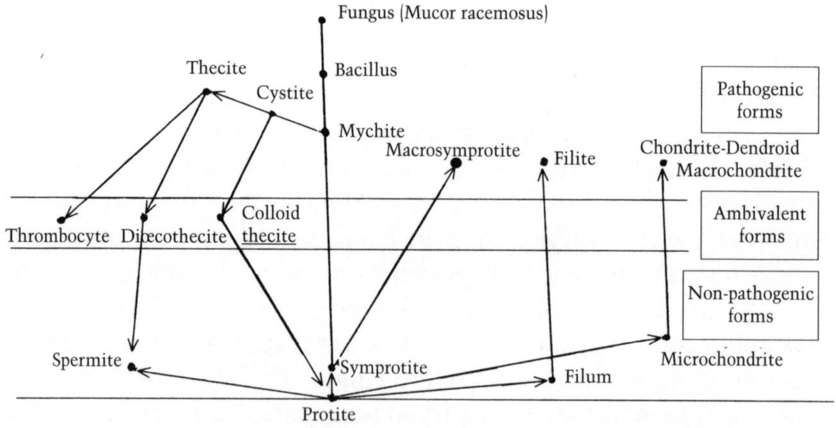

Fig.2: Upward development (Probaenogeny), modelled on the cyclode of Mucor racemosus Fresen - schematic representation.

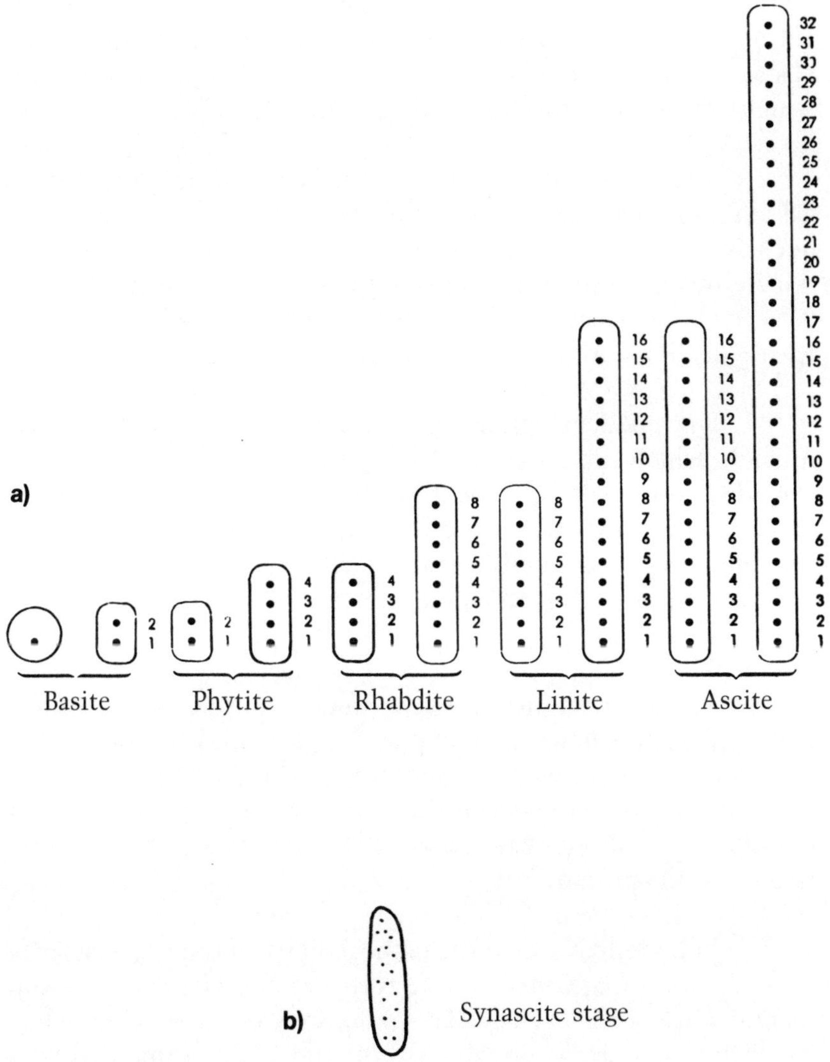

Fig.3: Probaenogeny in Leptotrichia buccalis
a) catatactic arrangement of nuclei; **b)** syntactic arrangement of nuclei
The pathogenicity increases with the number of nuclei or with their syntactic arrangement (from Akmon I).

At the end of a bacillus there are incomplete formations which are cut off; these are included among the growth forms of the bacterial stages. These particularly include the *gonidy*, a permanent stage which consists of a mychite with a firmer membrane.

The point of transition from the bacterial stages to the fungal stages is not fixed. At the highest point of a cyclode we frequently find fungal forms, as in the case of Mucor racemosus or Aspergillus niger. In other kinds of microbe the highest form may be at the basite stage (cocci) or at the chondrite stage. In these cases we are dealing with cyclodes which are incomplete.

Upward development (probaenogeny) is triggered by organic acids which are formed by the various growth forms of the cyclodes. In the case of Mucor racemosus it is lactic acid, in the case of Aspergillus niger it is citric acid, and in the case of Penicillium notatum it is penicillic acid. Enderlein called this dependence of probaenogeny upon the environmental pH the *"Fundamental Anartatic Law"*.

Moreover, in probaenogeny nuclear physics and quantum biological factors have a role to play. In quantum leaps the various growth forms merge with one another at lightning speed. Enderlein draws a comparison between this quantum biology and quantum physics. In the former case the smallest unit is the protite, in the latter it is the proton.

In Enderlein's view the pathogenicity of the various pathogenic agents is frequently only activated at one particular developmental stage of the cyclode. This stage may be situated anywhere along the cycle. However, this is not true of the primordial parasites or the primordial symbionts found in humans (various growth forms of the Mucor and Aspergillus cyclodes), which are constantly present within the organism. With the exception of the primitive stages (= symbionts) all the developmental stages are more or less pathogenic, depending on their *valency* (= stage of development).

Apart from the upward development mentioned above, Günther Enderlein also described further possibilities for development and transformation in micro-organisms (Table 1):

Table 1: Possibilities for development and transformation in micro-organisms

Probaenogeny	Upward development within the cyclode
Auxanogeny	Increasing development, asexual reproduction
Sexual reproduction	Union (copulation) of the spermite with the nuclei (mych) of all bacterial and fungal stages; transformation of these higher-valency forms into primitive forms.
Mochlosis	Blocking of probaenogeny
Mochlolysis	Clearing of the block (mochlosis)
Symplastism	Conglomeration of all growth forms of a cyclode into symplasts
Systatogeny	Unification of the protein colloids (protites), dehydration -> creation of dry protein forms (shock forms, permanent forms)

- These include so-called *auxanogeny*, i.e. increasing development (asexual reproduction), with which all bacteriologists are familiar. One example of this is the division of a mychite: two individual cells result from the division of the nucleus and the constriction of the cell (Fig.4).

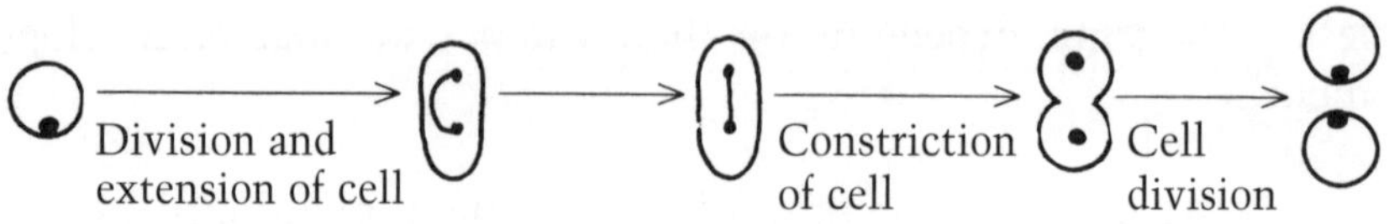

Fig.4: Division of a mychite (auxanogeny) (from Akmon I)

- As well as asexual reproduction, in the case of micro-organisms sexual reproduction also occurs. By this, Enderlein means the union (copulation) of the spermite with the nuclei (= mych) of all bacterial and fungal forms which form part of the same cycle. Copulation results in disintegration of the nucleus and the dismantling of the bacteria or fungi into primitive stages.
- In the case of mochlosis, upward development within the cyclode is inhibited. Development is halted at one particular stage. *Mochlolysis* is a freeing up of this block.
- By *systatogeny* Enderlein means the direct unification of protein colloids of the endobiont with other micro-organisms. The resulting shapes are dry protein forms, which may be observed in the blood in various illnesses. They are able to survive temperatures of up to 310 °C. The occurrence of chondrites at the corners characterises these sclerotic parasitic entities as permanent microbial forms. They include pseudo-crystals, sclerosymplasts, etc. (see Chapter 3).
- Symplastism denotes the conglomeration of various developmental forms of the cyclodes. The symplasts which are formed in this way make a highly significant contribution to dark field diagnosis (see Chapter 3).

3. Manifestations of Micro-organisms in the Blood

3.1 Blood plasma

3.1.1 Growth forms of the cyclodes

The human body plays host to primitive stages (symbionts) of the two mould species, Mucor racemosus and Aspergillus niger. The low-valency forms of Aspergillus primarily colonise the lymphatic system and connective tissue, whereas forms of Mucor occur in quantity in the blood and other cells of the body (Baum, 1987). However, this does not exclude the possibility of finding forms and shapes from the Aspergillus niger cyclode during a blood investigation, and these are highly significant in establishing a diagnosis (Tables 3 & 4). However, in the primitive stages it is not possible to draw a diagnostic distinction between these two original parasites.

In healthy blood only the non-pathogenic stages of Mucor racemosus are present, i.e. protite, filum, symprotite, spermite and microchondrite, the first two of these being invisible under the dark field microscope on account of their small size (Table 2). According to Enderlein symbionts are found in the blood plasma as well as in the blood cells. In the healthy organism, upward development into pathogenic forms is prevented by mochlosis.

As well as symbionts, platelets (thrombocytes) are found in the blood plasma, and according to Enderlein these form part of the Mucor racemosus cyclode. Thrombocytes, which have developed from thecites, provide us with an example of the ambivalence of the endobiont (Fig. 2). Orthodox opinion is that they are formed within bone marrow cells. Häfeli (1987) postulated that platelets come to maturity within erythrocytes and find their way into the blood plasma as required, or as a result of variations in pH values.

Table 2: Blood cells and micro-organisms in the blood (See illustrated section for size-comparison)

Blood cells	Erythrocyte Granulocyte Monocyte Lymphocyte	
Symbionts (Growth forms of primitive stages, non-pathogenic)	Protite Filum	Not visible under the dark field microscope owing to small size
	Spermite	Mobile defence corpuscle, degrades higher pathogenic forms of the endobiont.
	Symprotite Microchondrite	Low-valency forms of the endobiont
Parasitic growth forms of the primitive stage (pathogenic)	Macrosymprotite	Develops from symprotite by deposition of further protites
	Macrochondrite	Develops from microchondrite through upward development
	Sporoid symprotite	Symprotite whose protein occurs in a dry state owing to dehydration; permanent form, intensely luminous in dark field; partially coloured (yellowish -> upper abdominal indication, cornflower blue -> thyroid indication, green & white -> renal indication.)
	Filite	Develops from filum as a result of thickening

Table 2: Blood cells and micro-organisms in the blood (continued)

Parasitic growth forms of bacterial stages (pathogenic)	Mychite	Primary bacterial germ cell, with fixed nuclear wall
	Cystite	Spherical cell with a larger, polyvalent nucleus
	Thecite	Spherical cell with two or more nuclei
	Bacteria Bacilli or cocci a) Leptotrichia buccalis b) Mycobacterium tuberculosis c) Streptococci, Staphylococci	 Bacterial form of Mucor racemosus Bacterial form of Aspergillus niger Ultimate bacterial forms, basite stage
Ambivalent growth forms of bacterial stages	Thrombocyte	Platelet with 3-7 nuclei, blood coagulation
	Colloid thecite Diœcothecite	Forms which, as a result of spermite deficiency, may disintegrate, resulting in protite/spermite formation

Should the body's own symbiosis become unbalanced, then higher-valency, pathogenic growth forms occur, which are distinguishable in the blood plasma with particular clarity. In this case upward developments in various directions are possible.

a) Formation of parasitic growth forms of the primitive stages

If a symprotite enlarges, it can develop into a *macrosymprotite.* This is caused by an altered environment (Table 2).

The sporoid symprotite is a shape whose protein colloids are present in a dry state. Under the dark field microscope this form appears as a strongly refractive sphere.

The sporoid symprotite and the macrosymprotite may appear in both blood plasma and blood cells.

Table 3: Symplasts and sclerotic forms in the blood

Symplasts and sclerotic forms	Symplasts 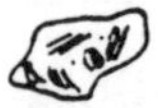	Conglomerations of various growth forms of cyclodes and of cell débris
	Sclerosymplast 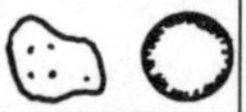	"Crystalline symplast", dry protein shape
	Pseudocrystals 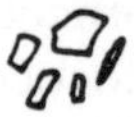	Creation from protein colloids of the endobiont and other microbes.
	Derosynacite 	Sclerotic shape, product of the synascite
	Drepanids 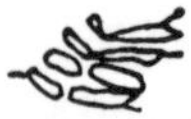	Small sickle-shaped discs of dry protein, arranged one behind the other
	Pteroharps 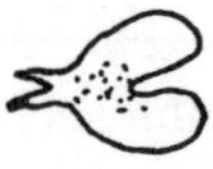	Fly-shaped grey objects consisting of sclerotic protein

Both forms are indicative of symbiotic disturbances in the body, the degree of pathogenicity rising with the increasing size (valency) of the symprotites. Thus the degree of overload may be observed from the relative size of the symprotites.

The filite is visible in the dark field and may develop from the filum as a result of pronounced thickening. Elevated filite formation in the blood plasma results in increased blood viscosity, leading to episodes of congestion and circulatory disturbances.

In chondrites we also find a higher developmental stage. In this case only the low-valency forms (microchondrites) are non-pathogenic. Their pathogenicity increases as they become thicker and larger, and countless forms exist.

b) Formation of parasitic growth forms of bacterial stages

As has already been described in Chapter 2, in the course of probaenogeny the protite is able to develop via the symprotite into the various bacterial stages. The mychite and thecite are pathogenic forms whose multiple presence indicates that the body's symbiosis is off-track. If sufficient spermites are present in the blood, it is possible to dismantle these growth forms.

The presence of Leptotrichia buccalis bacilli in the blood is indicative of an overload from the Mucor cyclode (see Chapter 4). The degree of overload rises with the number of bacilli observed and also with their length (number of nuclei) and thickness. Bacteria whose nuclei are arranged three-dimensionally (synascites) indicate a higher level of pathogenicity than bacilli, which have a linear nuclear arrangement (ascites)*. The origins of bacilli in the blood lie mainly in the so-called "marginal granules" (symprotites) of erythrocytes (see Chapter 3.2).

[*Transl. note: Wherever the word 'ascites' occurs in this text, it is as the plural of 'ascite' (two syllables) and has no connection with the English medical term 'ascites' (three syllables) which denotes fluid accumulation in the abdomen.]

In the blood of tuberculosis patients, Mycobacterium tuberculosis bacilli only occur during the haematogenic scattering stage. This can be demonstrated either directly by fluorescent microscopy (Ziehl-Neelsen's stain) or by a bacteriological culture from sputum, gastric juices, urine etc. Streptococci and staphylococci can only be demonstrated in the blood in septic cases. Classic symptoms of this severe illness are high fever, shivering fits, and a haemorrhagic diathesis. Because of their shape, the mychite chains of Leptotrichia buccalis which are occasionally seen in dark field microscopy may easily be confused with various kinds of streptococcus (p.63). However, it is possible to differentiate on the basis of the individual patient's symptoms, or of a culture.

c) Formation of ambivalent growth forms of bacterial stages

During upward development within the cyclode ambivalent growth forms may come into being, such as thrombocytes, colloid thecites and diœcothecites (Fig. 2). As already mentioned in Chapter 2, thrombocytes develop from thecites. The number of nuclei of platelets generally ranges between 3 and 7. Pathogenic forms with numerous nuclei and fila may result from enlargement or conglomeration of several thrombocytes. Such degenerate thrombocytes indicate that the body's endobiont is off-track. (Chap.4, table 4).

Another developmental form of the thecite is the *diœcothecite*, as described by Enderlein, which is filled with numerous tiny nuclei (micromych). It consists of a thin membrane, whose outer surface is covered with many short, fine fila. The size of a diœcothecite varies from that of a thrombocyte up to that of an erythrocyte, with both oval and round forms occurring. In the event of a deficiency of symbionts, diœcothecites may disintegrate into a large number of spermites. Thus they constitute a reservoir of spermites which may be released as required. Particularly in the case of the seriously ill, the presence of diœcothecites in the dark field blood picture indicates that the body is prepared for defensive action. The number of these regulators in the blood is variable. Enderlein quotes percentages of up to 100% of the erythrocyte count. Diœcothecites occur particularly at points in the blood picture which indicate infective foci (see illustrated section).

The *colloid-thecite* is a grey, spherical shape with a delicate sheath and consists of a conglomeration of protein colloids. This shape, as described by Enderlein, lacks a nucleus and develops either from symprotites, sporoid symprotites or from cystites. In the latter case this is the result of disintegration of the polyvalent nucleus into protein colloids. The colloid-thecite varies in size between that of a thrombocyte and that of an erythrocyte. Large quantities of microsymprotites can be released if required as a result of the colloid-thecite's membrane bursting. These serve to dismantle higher-valency pathogenic forms. The presence of colloid-thecites in the blood picture indicates that the body is prepared for defensive action.

d) Formation of fungal stages

The culmination of the cyclode - the fungal Mucor racemosus - only colonises the body after death. In moribund patients one may occasionally observe transitional forms between the bacterial and fungal stages.

3.1.2 Symplasts and sclerotic forms

Symplasts are conglomerations of various growth forms of the cyclodes, including tissue residues from blood cells and toxins. The formation of symplasts means that pathogenic forms in the organism are withdrawn from circulation. Symplastism flourishes in an alkaline environment. If the body's own defence mechanism is functioning, then a dismantling of these conglomerations is possible. The symplast either dissolves into low-valency chondrites and symprotites or is dismantled by granulocytes (p. 72) (Arnoul, 1992). The number and size of the symplasts is an indication of the degree of overload in the individual patient.

The sclerotic parasitic shapes include *"crystalline symplasts" (sclerosymplasts), pseudocrystals, pteroharps, drepanids, derosynascites*, and many others. Enderlein was the first to describe these shapes, which have their origin in the process of *systatogeny*, i.e. the coming together of protein colloids (protites) of the endobiont and other parasites. In such sclerotic shapes, as a result of dehydration, the colloids occur in the form of dry protein. They are capable of surviving temperatures of up to 310°C. Enderlein described them as shock forms or permanent forms. The shape and colour of sclerosymplasts are frequently an indication of the overload of certain organs (Table 3). The colloid nature of these shapes is clearly identifiable by the presence of chondrites at the corners and edges.

The highly pathogenic *derosynascite* has its origin in a bacillus, as a result of the disintegration of the primary nuclei into numerous smaller nuclei (cryptomych). These cryptomychs form clusters on the outer membrane, forming black, sclerotic thorns. Derosynascites are found particularly in cases of serious disease, such as cancer, AIDS, Hodgkin's, etc.

Drepanids consist of small sickle-shaped discs of dry protein, arranged one behind the other. These sclerotic, parasitic shapes may easily be distinguished from similar inorganic forms by the chondrite processes at their edges. Drepanids may occur in various chronic diseases.

According to Enderlein, *pteroharps* occur particularly in cases of more advanced endobiosis and of the consequent diseases, such as cancer, benign tumours, intestinal haemorrhage, asthma, etc. Enderlein derived the name of this formation, which is composed of sclerosed protein from living colloids, from its function and shape as a "winged robber". He suspected that pteroharps require protein from erythrocytes for their construction. These fly-like shapes originate from protein colloids of either Mucor racemosus or Aspergillus niger. In size they are at least half the diameter of an erythrocyte. Under the dark field microscope pteroharps are visible as delicate grey shapes.

3.2 Erythrocytes

Healthy erythrocytes are only infested by small numbers of low-valency growth forms of Mucor racemosus (symprotites, microchondrites). In the event of symbiosis being disturbed there is an initial increase in the number of these non-pathogenic primitive stages. Following this purely numerical increase, the first higher-valency forms (sporoid symprotites, macrosymprotites) appear in the red corpuscles, with a rise in pathogenicity according to valency and size.

As the blood cells shrivel - a process which takes several hours - so the microbes present in the erythrocytes find their way into the plasma, provided there is no block in operation. The valency and number of the growth forms released depend on the nature and severity of the patient's illness. If the organism is under heavy stress, the forms entering the blood plasma will be of predominantly high valency (bacteria, macrochondrites); if the stress is lower, they will be symprotites or low-valency chondrites. If a block exists, the microbes remain within the blood cells.

Depending on the valency and the degree of infestation of the erythrocytes, various phenomena may be observed (Table 4).

Table 4: Interpretation of blood pictures under the dark field microscope

a) Blood plasma

Forms/Phenomena	Description/ Depiction	Cause/Diagnosis
Protite veil	Greyish-white veil	pH value of blood too high -> disintegration of symbionts into smallest units (protites)
Filite formation	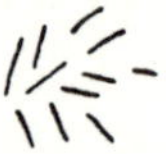	Endobiosis, Mucor cyclode off-track ->congestions, circulatory disturbances / stress level dependent on strength and frequency of occurrence of filites and on their distribution within the blood picture
Spermites/ Symprotites[1]	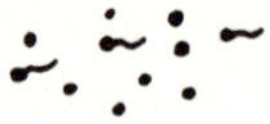	Statement regarding body's readiness for defence against pathogenic forms, high level of activity -> virulence, infection; low level of activity -> symbiontic weakness of defence.
Macrosymprotites/ Sporoid symprotites		Increased occurrence in blood plasma -> disturbance of symbiosis, disease process (partially indicative of increase in protein supply); see Table 2 re. coloured symprotites
Free chondrites	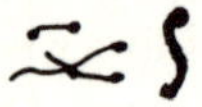	Non-pathogenic microchondrites, macro-chondrites -> disease
Mychites, Thecites		Occurrence in large numbers -> disturbed symbiosis

[1] The spermite's flagellum is so thin that it is not detectable under dark field microscope.

Table 4: Interpretation of blood pictures under the dark field microscope (continued)

a) Blood plasma

Forms/Phenomena	Description/ Depiction	Cause/Diagnosis
Thrombocytes	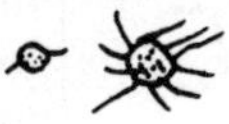	Platelets with 3-7 nuclei; conglomeration and enlargement of thrombocytes -> congestions and circulatory disturbances
Colloid thecite	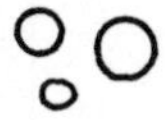	Ambivalent form of endobiont, presence -> organism prepared for defence
Diœcothecite	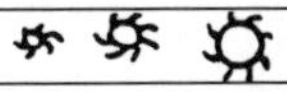	See Colloid thecite
Bacteria	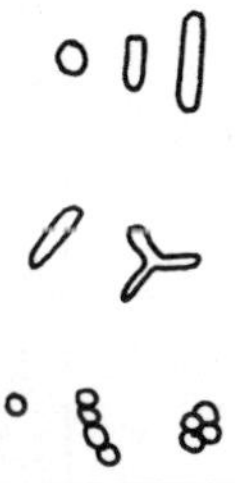	Leptotrichia buccalis -> with increased occurrence, diseases of the Mucor cyclode; degree of pathogenicity dependent on number of nuclei, i.e. length of bacilli, with synascites being more pathogenic than ascites.
Symplasts	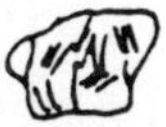	Indication of a shift in blood pH value towards alkaline, degree of overload dependent on frequency of occurrence and on size; light-coloured symplasts -> overload with Mucor, i.e. overload with parasitic forms from Mucor cyclode; dark-coloured symplasts -> overload with Aspergillus, i.e. overload with parasitic forms from Aspergillus cyclode; circulation of blood inhibited

Table 4: Interpretation of blood pictures under the dark field microscope (continued)

a) Blood plasma

Forms/Phenomena	Description/ Depiction	Cause/Diagnosis
Sclerotic forms "crystalline symplast" (sclerosymplast)	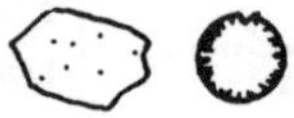	Inhibited blood flow; overload in various areas according to colour (green -> genito-urinary tract and kidneys; yellow and brown -> upper abdomen, liver, gallbladder; cornflower blue -> thyroid
Pseudocrystals	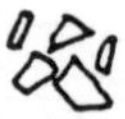	According to shape and colour, indicative of overload of various areas; yellow and brown -> upper abdomen
Derosynascite		In cases of severe chronic disease (Hodgkins, AIDS, leukæmia), highly pathogenic form
Drepanids	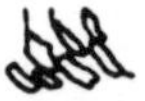	In cases of various chronic diseases
Pteroharps	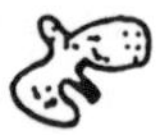	In cases of various chronic diseases, consist of colloids of Mucor racemosus or Aspergillus niger

b) Infestation of erythrocytes

Forms/Phenomena	Description/ Depiction	Cause/Diagnosis
Agglutination of erythrocytes: rouleaux formation	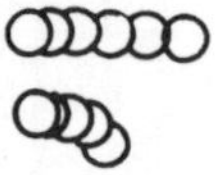	Endobiosis -> congestions, circulatory disturbances, curved rouleaux (according to Prigge) -> intestinal overload

Table 4: Interpretation of blood pictures under the dark field microscope (continued)

b) Infestation of erythrocytes

Forms/Phenomena	Description/ Depiction	Cause/Diagnosis
Honeycomb arrangement	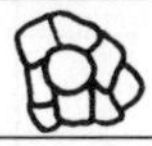	Endobiosis -> thrombi of erythrocytes
Anisocytosis	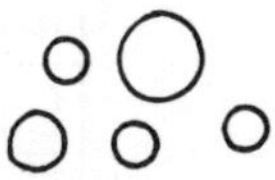	Difference in size of erythrocytes as a result of pathogenic action of the endobiont e.g. in anæmia
Poikilocytosis		Changes in form of erythrocytes resulting from action of endobiont
Erythrocytes with central shimmering	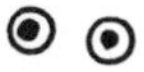	Lowest stage of endobiosis, mild patho-genicity
Lemon-shaped erythrocytes	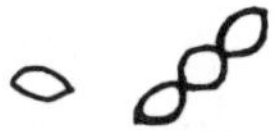	Singly or concatenated -> indicative of hepatic overload
Cells resembling targets		Endobiontic overload
Erythrocytes with symprotites or chondrites at edges	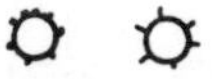	
Reticulocytes	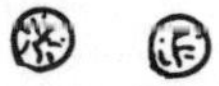	
Thorn-apple shapes	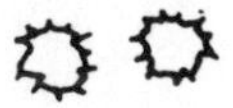	These develop from a shrinking process, low-valency infestation where processes are numerous and thin, high degree of endobiosis where processes are few and thick
Erythrocytes with sporoid symprotites	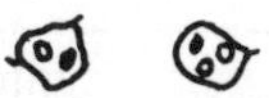	Degree of endobiosis depends on size and number of sporoid symprotites, as well as on number of affected erythrocytes
Erythrocytes with chondrites	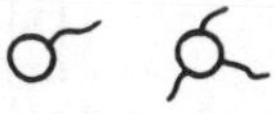	Endobiosis in acute and chronic diseases

Table 4: Interpretation of blood pictures under the dark field microscope (continued)

b) Infestation of erythrocytes

Forms/Phenomena	Description/ Depiction	Cause/Diagnosis
Erythrocytes with tubular excrescences	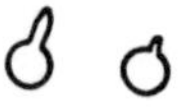	Development of bacterial forms from fixed-wall symprotites of erythrocytes; high degree of endobiosis
Erythrocytes with vacuoles		Consumption of substance of erythrocytes by endobionts, appearance of vacuoles immediately after decrease -> high degree of endobiosis
Sclerotic changes in erythrocytes	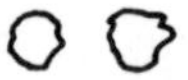	Heavy endobiontic overload
Disintegration of erythrocytes	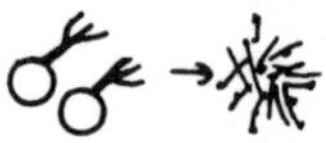	Disintegration of erythrocytes into chondrite-dendroids -> severe chronic disease
		Disintegration of erythrocytes into fragments -> severe chronic disease or overload with infective foci

c) Infestation of leucocytes

Forms/Phenomena	Description/ Depiction	Cause/Diagnosis
Infestaton of leucocytes (nucleus and plasma)	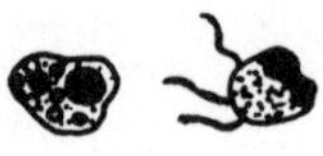	Infestation with high-valency chondrite forms, thecites, sporoid symprotites or thrombocytes, degree of overload depends on valency and on number of leucocytes affected -> cellular defence weakened

c) Infestation of leucocytes (continued)

Forms/Phenomena	Description/ Depiction	Cause/Diagnosis
Leucocytes with pseudopodiae	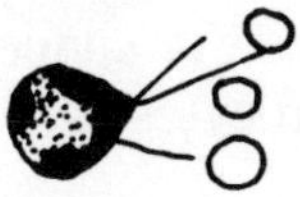	Leucocytes severely infested with parasitic forms, pseudopodiae = chondrite-dendroids -> cellular defence weakened
Disintegration of leucocytes and lymphocytes	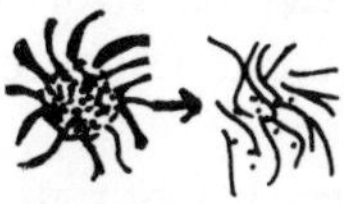	Parasitic growth forms of the endobiont (chondrite-dendroids) with stringy excrescences, followed by disintegration of leucocytes -> defence extinguished, seen in pictures of severe illness
Disintegration of leucocytes into capsules of spermites and symprotites	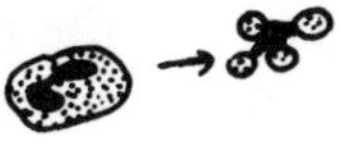	Activation of defence mechanism in order to eliminate pathogenic growth forms -> formation of spermites and symprotites (Arnoul, 1992)
Increase in leucocytes and lymphocytes, appearance of immature forms		Leucocytosis, in cases of leukæmia and infectious diseases etc.

The lowest stage of endobiosis is recognizable under the dark field microscope by a *central shimmering* of the erythrocytes. Presumably this phenomenon may be attributed to a purely numerical increase in primitive stages of Mucor racemosus.

Lemon-shaped erythrocytes are indicative of hepatic overload. This particular form results from endobiontic action. When the blood picture is turbulent, the red corpuscles may temporarily assume a lemon-shaped form, so long as a flow is present. In these cases it is necessary to check whether the lemon-shape persists once the blood picture has calmed down. Pear-shaped erythrocytes occur particularly when the spleen is under stress. In patients with a severely enlarged spleen the blood picture may exhibit over 50% of these characteristically shaped red corpuscles.

Reticulocytes are red blood corpuscles containing chondrite-dendroids. According to Enderlein there is an increase in reticulocytes in cases of heavy metal intoxication inter alia.

So far as *Heinz bodies* are concerned, these are parasitic symprotites within the erythrocytes.

In the case of *target cells* (cells resembling shooting targets) there is an unequal distribution of hæmoglobin in the erythrocytes owing to pathogenic endobiontic forms.

Thorn apple shapes result from an increase in number and size of symprotites internally. The surface of such an endobiotically infested red corpuscle is covered with fila and chondrites. The degree of infestation depends on the relative size of the symprotites. Large, high-valency symprotites cause the erythrocyte to shrivel, with a small number of thick processes as on a thorn apple, whereas small, low-valency symprotites result in a profusion of thin processes.

The appearance of *sporoid symprotites in the red corpuscles* indicates a further increase in valency of the endobiontic infestation. In cases of serious disease (cancer, etc.) the size of the high-valency symprotite granules may amount to as much as one quarter or one third of the erythrocyte's diameter. Moreover, the number of affected erythrocytes is crucial in determining the degree of infestation.

Erythrocytes with vacuoles, which appear as soon as the blood sample has been taken, are indicative of a severe endobiontic overload. The development of the vacuoles results from the consumption of the substance of the red corpuscles by parastic growth forms of Mucor racemosus.

In cases of severe chronic disease, bacilli of *Leptotrichia buccalis* may develop from marginal symprotites (Schilling's marginal granules). This process was first described by Enderlein. The symprotite situated on the membrane of the erythrocyte deposits numerous protites for the formation of cell plasma (Fig.1). Thus a mychite is produced, in which the original symprotite adopts the role of primary nucleus (mych). Finally the bacillus is formed, as a result of nuclear division and extension, detaching itself from the erythrocyte as the process continues. Symprotites of various coccal forms, which have attached themselves to the membrane of the erythrocyte, may similarly form chains or clusters (streptococci or staphylococci).

Erythrocytes with *chondritic outgrowths* occur in a wide variety of diseases (acute infections, chronic diseases).

The disintegration of erythrocytes into *chondrite-dendroids* indicates a high degree of endobiosis. The same is true of an increased incidence of *blood shadows*, i.e. red corpuscles which have lost their hæmoglobin. Where there is an overload of infective foci, it is common for erythrocytes to disintegrate into smaller fragments.

Agglutination of red corpuscles in fasting blood samples (rouleaux formation, honeycomb arrangement) occurs as a consequence of a rise in the valency of chondrite forms which are present in the blood cells. These grow out from the erythrocytes. Agglutination takes place as a result of the union of chondrites from various corpuscles. According to Prigge (1990) rouleaux with a curved shape are indicative of intestinal overload.

The increase in valency of the endobiont is a response to environmental change within the body. Causes of such change include individual predisposition, a protein-rich diet, unhealthy lifestyle, stress, emotional pressures, etc. For the erythrocytes, agglutination or a change in shape results in restriction of both functional ability and mobility. The consequences of this are circulatory disturbances, congestions, a reduced oxygen supply to the cells and hyperacidity of the connective tissue.

3.3 Leucocytes

The white corpuscles too may exhibit varying stages of infestation. A disturbance in symbiosis within the organism is accompanied by a rise in valency of the symprotites in the granulocytes, monocytes and lymphocytes. Finally these symprotites will develop into sporoid symprotites, chondrites, thecites, thrombocytes or bacteria, all of which may be clearly recognised under the dark field microscope.

The leucocyte attempts to rid itself of these parasitic elements. Enderlein describes this process as follows:

"It is unbelievably easy to see numerous erythrocytes helpfully approaching the leucocytes and lymphocytes which have become severely infested with endobiontic symprotites. They surge towards the sick white blood cell, taking the parasitic symprotites upon themselves, frequently stuffing themselves full" (end of quote). In this case the transfer of the symprotites is effected either directly or via pseudopodiæ which, according to Enderlein, are the equivalent of the chondrite-dendroids of the endobiont.

As the valency rises, tree- or cord-like projections may grow out from the leucocytes (chondrite-dendroids), finally resulting in the disintegration of the white corpuscles. During the formation of these parasitic, highly pathogenic forms, the substance of the affected white corpuscle is either partially or wholly consumed.

Dendroid disintegration of leucocytes and lymphocytes occurs in various severe chronic diseases (ulcus cruris, cancer, etc.)

Increased presence of leucocytes results in leucocytosis.

4 Disease Pictures and their Place within the Cyclodes

In ancient times, the diseases of human beings were attributed to changes in the humours of the body. This *humoral pathology*, which had its origins in the Babylonian and Egyptian cultures, was adopted by Hippocrates (460-359 BC) and further developed by Hahnemann (1755-1843). Orthodox medicine, on the other hand, is based on *cellular pathology*, as postulated by Virchow (1821-1902). This states that the cause of every illness is to be sought in a disturbance of individual cells.

In parallel to this, in bacteriology Pasteur's starting point of monomorphism became generally accepted. Diseases of microbial origin were allotted specific causative agents (see Chapter 1). Enderlein returned to Béchamp's pleomorphistic view and the thinking of humoral pathology. He provided proof that, in the bodies of vertebrates, micro-organisms (symbionts) occur, which belong to the cyclodes of Mucor racemosus and Aspergillus niger. On account of changes in the physical environment, these symbionts can develop into parasitic forms, should the body's defence mechanism fail.

Within the organism, upward development in the Mucor cyclode brings about an increase in thickness of the blood, for instance, resulting from filite formation and agglutination of erythrocytes. Enderlein described this process as a congestive tendency, or *endobiosis*. Where there is endobiosis, the blood cells have become infested with parasitic growth forms (see Chapter 3). The thickening of the blood leads to circulatory disturbances with their consequences, such as venous congestion, thromboses and strokes (see Table 5).

Mucor racemosus cyclode		
Mucor racemosus cyclode	Aspergillus niger cyclode	Cyclodes culminating in various types of coccus
Venous diseases Disturbances in arterial circulation Apoplexy Hearing loss Insidious occlusion of the vessels Thrombocytopænia Cervical syndrome Osteomyelosclerosis Certain forms of rheumatism	Bronchitis Tuberculosis Croupy cough Ankylosing spondylitis Arthrosis and arthritis of the joints Cancers AIDS Certain forms of rheumatism Diseases of the thyroid gland	Inflammations Osteomyelitis Certain forms of rheumatism Gout Sinusitis Infective foci

The higher-valency growth forms of the Aspergillus cyclode may provoke disturbances in the calcium metabolism or in the citric acid cycle of the cells. They result in diseases of the respiratory tract and the skeletal system, and also in tuberculosis, cancer, etc. In such diseases, particularly in cancer, parasitic forms of the Mucor cyclode are always involved in the pathogenic process. This is owing to the fact that both cyclodes are linked and, in the rarest cases, are totally portrayable so far as diagnosis and treatment are concerned. There is a further derivative of the Aspergillus niger cyclode, which culminates in the fungus Penicillium notatum.

Diseases of coccal origin may be successfully treated with low-valency forms of Penicillium notatum. Such diseases particularly include inflammations, sinusitis, osteo-myelitis and certain forms of rheumatism.

Regarding chronic diseases Enderlein finally speaks of a bipolar pair of forceps, embracing the complex of *endobiontic diseases* (Mucor racemosus) and the *tubercular complex* (Aspergillus niger).

Disease pictures and their place within the Cyclodes

The allocation of diseases to particular cyclodes may be regarded as a rough guideline. In most cases several cyclodes are involved. For this reason, in treatment, it is not possible to make a precise delimitation.

5 Interpretation of Blood Pictures under the Dark Field Microscope

In dark field diagnosis success or failure are dependent on various factors. These include meticulous care in making up the slide preparation, as well as a purposeful and systematic evaluation. A detailed description of the procedure follows.

Taking the blood sample

As a rule the sample is taken from the patient's finger-tip when the stomach is empty. Having pricked the finger-tip with a sterile lancet, the first and second drops to emerge are wiped off with a swab. Now, without squeezing the finger at all, a little blood is taken with a clean cover glass from the surface of the third drop. If at all possible any contact of the cover glass with the finger-tip must be avoided, so as to prevent any possible contamination of the slide preparation. Avoiding any air-bubbles, the cover glass is carefully placed on the slide of the microscope. Before use the slide has been wiped with a clean linen cloth. The amount of blood applied is important in arriving at an optimum interpretation of the blood picture. As a rule of thumb: once the drop has been placed on the slide, $^{2}/_{3}$ to $^{3}/_{4}$ of the cover glass at the most should be covered.

Causes of errors

- Utilization of peripheral blood (puncture too shallow) -> changes in the blood components, e.g. severely deformed erythrocytes (thorn-apple shapes) owing to the oxygen in the air

- Consumption of food before the sample is taken -> rouleaux formation of erythrocytes or lemon-shaped erythrocytes; -> increased quantity and activity of the symbionts present in the blood plasma (spermites, symprotites), occurrence of chylomicrons etc.

- Use of chemical agents (alcohol, etc.) to clean microscope slides and cover glasses or to sterilise the finger-tip -> changes in the blood components.

Dark field microscopy

As soon as the sample has been taken the blood picture should be examined, initially for an overview, i.e. using the lowest degree of magnification. It is recommended first of all to scan the whole slide preparation from top to bottom, and then from left to right, so as to gain an overall impression. The marginal areas of the preparation are excluded from the interpretation, since there will be changes in the blood cells there owing to the action of oxygen in the air. Even with this low magnification, it is still possible to make judgements regarding:

- Homogeneity or heterogeneity of the blood smear. Are there (e.g.) any dark spots (indications of infective foci)?
- Number of erythrocytes, possible rouleaux formations or honeycomb arrangements (agglutination);
- Number of leucocytes;
- Number, size, form and colour of symplasts and sclerotic shapes

The same procedure is now repeated with a more powerful degree of magnification (1:1200), paying particular attention to the following criteria:

- *The red blood picture*: shape and functional ability of erythrocytes, microbial infestation of erythrocytes. What percentage of the red corpuscles is infested? Which parasitic forms occur in the erythrocytes?
- *The white blood picture*: shape, functional ability and quality of the leucocytes and lymphocytes and their microbial infestation. Which parasitic forms occur in the leucocytes? Are immature leucocytes present? Are any disintegrated white corpuscles present?
- *The blood plasma*:

a) The various forms of the endobiont which occur in it, their frequency of occurrence and their activity;

b) Number, shape and size of thrombocytes;
c) Composition and colour of the symplasts;
d) Composition, shape and frequency of occurrence of sclerotic formations

It is recommended that the blood be observed over the space of several hours or days, since the products of disintegration and its duration are of great importance in establishing the diagnosis (Dr. Baum, oral communication). According to Prigge (1990), disintegration of the blood after 1.5 - 2 hours is a sign of severe illness, whereas a slow disintegration over 48 - 72 hours indicates an absence of chronic disease. However, this is only valid where factors such as temperature etc. remain constant. In high external temperatures the disintegration time is considerably shortened.

If a blood sample is observed over several hours or days, the following factors are also decisive in the interpretation:
- How rapidly do the erythrocytes change? When, for instance, do thorn-apple shapes, erythrocytes with vacuoles or with chondrite-dendroids appear?
- Is any disintegration of erythrocytes or leucocytes present? What products of disintegation appear?
- Are higher-valency forms entering the plasma? If not, either a block or a slight degree of overload is present. What growth forms are being released from the blood cells (symprotites, chondrites, bacteria)?
- Are certain phenomena of a temporary or permanent nature? Rouleaux, for instance, may dissolve after a while. In that case the overload is temporary, i.e. an acute episode. If there is no dissolution, we are dealing with a chronic process. In this case, after a few hours, agglutination may be aggravated.
- How long does it take for filites to appear in the plasma?
- What colours appear at the margins of the preparation as it dries out? According to Prigge (1990) a red margin (hæmoglobin leakage) indicates a paratubercular illness, and green indicates an overload in the genito-urinary tract.

When interpreting blood pictures it must be taken into account that, in cases of chronic disease, initial observations under the dark field microscope sometimes lead to no result as the pathogens have manifested themselves in the blood and body cells. Such a block may be dissolved by means of an appropriate stimulative treatment (Arnoul, 1992). In no case should the practitioner rely exclusively on dark field microscopy, but should always make every attempt to reach a summative diagnosis.

Native Blood Investigation by Dark Field Microscopy

First Name & Family Name ______________________ D.o.b. ________
Address ____
Diagnosis ____

Blood plasma

Protite veil	Yes/No
Filite formation	+/++/+++* Distribution over whole blood picture Yes/No
Symbionts (Spermites & Symprotites)	Frequency and Activity +/++/+++*
Macrosymprotites	Yes/No, Frequency
Sporoid Symprotites	Yes/No, Frequency
Free Chondrites	Yes/No, Frequency and Valency
Mychites	Yes/No, Frequency
Thecites	Yes/No, Frequency
Thrombocytes	Number, Enlarged/Conglomerations
Colloid Thecites	Yes/No, Frequency
Diœcothecites	Yes/No, Frequency

Bacteria

Cocci	Yes/No, Frequency
Leptotrichia buccalis	Yes/No, Frequency, Stages (Ascites/Synascites)
Sclerothrix tuberculosis	Yes/No, Frequency, Stages
Symplasts	Frequency (1-5), Size & Colour
Sclerosymplasts	Frequency (1-5), Size & Colour
Pseudocrystals	Frequency, Colour
White Crystals	Frequency
Sclerotic parasitic formations	Forms (e.g. Drepanids, Pteroharps)

---

* + = weak, ++ = medium, +++ = strong

<u>Erythrocytes</u>

Agglutination

Honeycombed	Yes/No
Bank rolls	+/++/+++
Anisocytosis	Yes/No

Poikilocytosis

Valency:	Forms (e.g. thorn-apple, erythrocytes with vacuoles, etc.)
Strength	+/++/+++
Sclerotic changes in erythrocytes	Yes/No
Disintegration	Yes/No

<u>Leucocytes</u>

Number of leucocytes	Increased/Normal/Low

Endobiosis of leucocytes

Valency (Granulocytes, Monocytes)	Forms (e.g. infestation of granulocytes and monocytes with sporoid symprotites, chron-drite-dendroids, thrombocytes, bacteria)
Strength	+/++/+++

Endobiosis of Lymphocytes

Valency	Forms (e.g. infestation of granulocytes and monocytes with sporoid symprotites, chron drite-dendroids, thrombocytes)
Strength	+/++/+++

Disintegration of leucocytes into:

a) Spermite capsules	Yes/No
b) Chondrite-Dendroids	Yes/No

Overall interpretation ____

____

Remarks ____

____

Illustrated part

The following photographs were taken with the help of a Zeiss axioscope with darkfield condenser and connected Nikon miniature camera (magnification 1:1200).

The following slide films were used: Ektachrome 200 and 400.

On account of the strong magnification, the chosen illustrations are only small details which generally do not represent the total blood picture.

The illustrated darkfield phenomenons were usually photographed at least 15 minutes after having made the preparation. If this period of time was passed, a remark was made in the texts of the picture.

A burdening of the organism with parasitic growth forms of the Mucor racemosus and Aspergillus niger cyclodes will be shortly described in the following as „Mucor burden" resp. „Aspergillus burden". However, these two terms do not refer to the culminations of the two cyclodes, namely the fungal phases.

The same is valid for the terming of the symplasts („Mucor-" or „Aspergillus-symplast").

Bestandteile des Blutes – Blutzellen

Patient: W., geb. 1960
Diagnose: Chronische Sinusitis

Components of the blood – blood cells

Patient: W., born 1960
Diagnosis: Chronic sinusitis

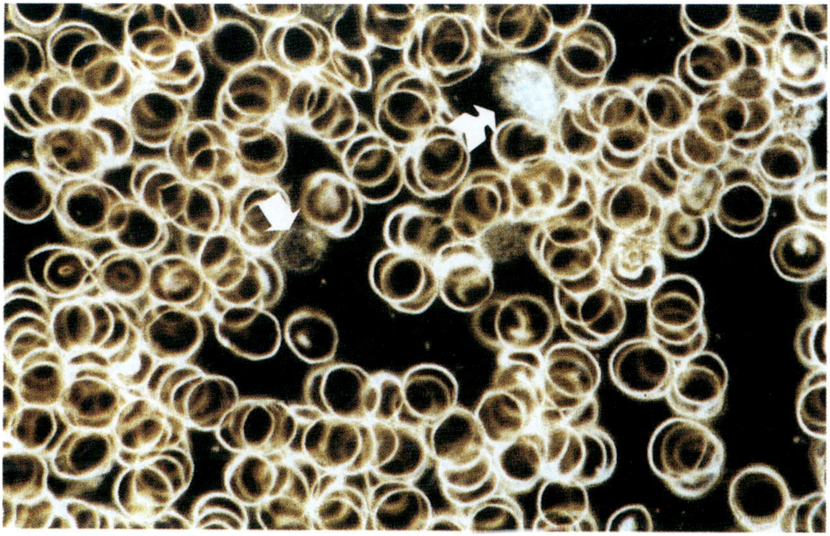

Aufnahme von: 9/1992 – Photo taken: 9/1992

Bewertung: Leichte Agglutination der Erythrozyten; geringe Anzahl von Symbionten im Plasma.

➽ Granulozyt ➡ Lymphozyt

Evaluation: Slight agglutination of the erythrocytes; small number of symbionts in the plasma.

➽ granulocyte ➡ lymphocyte

Blutplasma

Filitbildung

Patientin: R., geb. 1956
Diagnose: Varizen, Durchblutungsstörungen in beiden Beinen, Lumbago

Blood plasma

Filit formation

Patient (female): R., born 1956
Diagnosis: Varicose veins, disturbances of blood supply in both legs, lumbago

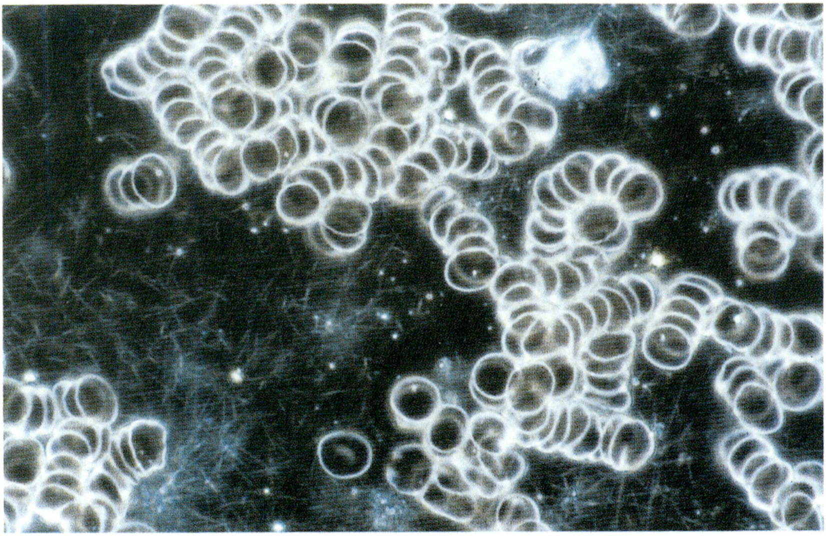

Aufnahme von: 10/1990 – Photo taken: 10/1990

Bewertung: Filitbildung – erhöhte Fibrinbildung, „Mucor-Belastung"; Agglutination der Erythrozyten – Endobiose, Stauungen; gebogene Geldrollen – nach Prigge (1990) Darmbelastung

Evaluation: Filit formation – increased fibrin formation, „Mucor burden"; agglutination of the erythrocytes – endobiosis, congestions; curved coin rolls – according to Prigge (1990) intestinal stress

Symbionten (Spermite/Symprotite)

Patient: J., geb. 1937
Diagnose: Akute Bronchitis

Symbionts (spermits/symprotits)

Patient: J., born 1937
Diagnosis: Acute bronchititis

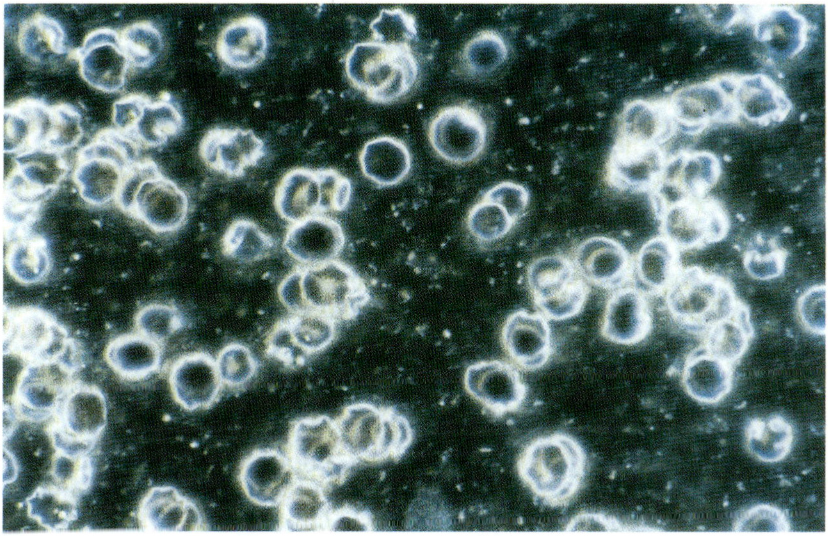

Aufnahme von: 5/1989 – Photo taken: 5/1989

Bewertung: Hohe Spermit-/Symprotitaktivität im Plasma – Virulenz, Infektion; Erythrozyten verformt – endobiontische Belastung aufgrund der akuten Infektion (1 h nach Blutentnahme).

Evaluation: High activities of spermits/symprotits in the plasma – virulency, infection; deformed erythrocytes – endobiontic burden on account of the acute infection (one hour after taking of blood sample).

Patient: R., geb. 1926
Diagnose: Tumor im linken Auge (Ca)

Patient (female): R., born 1926
Diagnosis: Tumor in the left eye (ca)

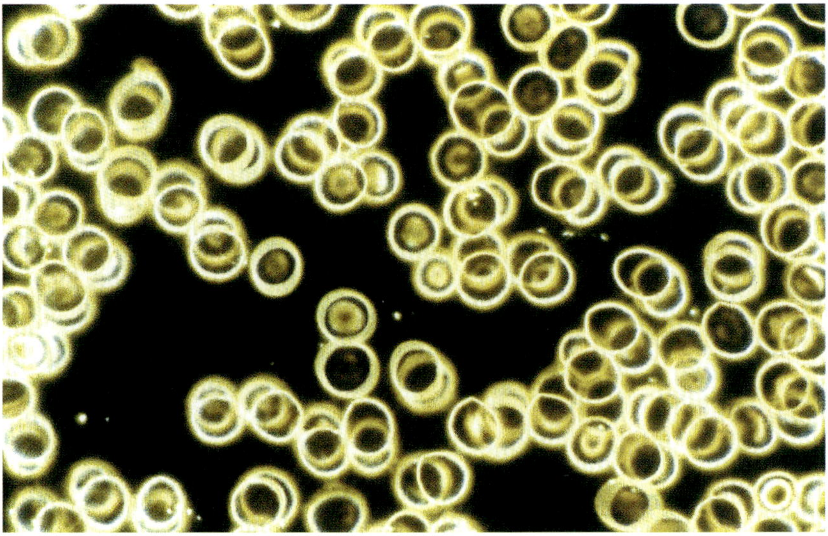

Aufnahme von: 8/1992 – Photo taken: 8/1992

Bewertung: Geringe Anzahl von Symbionten im Plasma – Immunsystem (symbiontische Abwehr) geschwächt, zentrales Flimmern in den Erythrozyten.

Evaluation: Small number of symbionts in the plasma – immunological system (symbiontic defence) weakened, central glimmer in the erythrocytes.

Sporoide Symprotite

Patientin: S., geb. 1956
Diagnose: Intoxikation mit Holzschutzmittel, chronische Enteritis, Hyperthyreose

Sporoid symprotits

Patient (female): S., born 1956
Diagnosis: Intoxication with wood preservation, chronic enteritis, hyperthyreosis

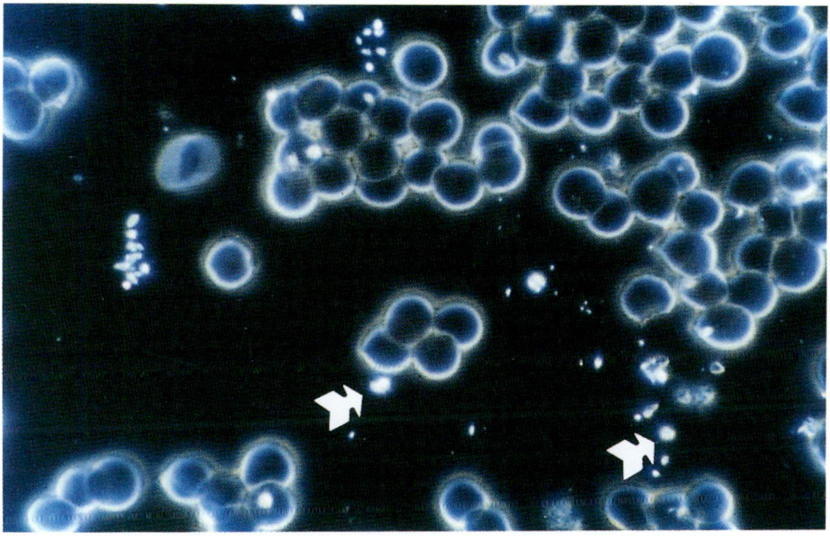

Aufnahme von: 12/1988 – Photo taken: 12/1988

Bewertung: ➽ Zahlreiche sporoide Symprotite im Plasma – Aufwärtsentwicklung der Symprotite zu pathogenen Formen, Symbiosestörung; Agglutination der Erythrozyten – endobiontische Belastung; einige zitronenförmige Erythrozyten – Leberbelastung; starke Lumineszenz der Erythrozytenmembranen – nach Prigge (1990) Energieschwäche der Erythrozyten.

Evaluation: ➽ Numerous sporoid symprotits in the plasma – upward development of the symprotits into pathogenic forms; disturbance of symbiosis: agglutination of the erythrocytes – endobiontic burden; some lemonshaped erythrocytes – liver burden; strong luminescence of the membranes of the erythrocytes – according to Prigge (1990) weakness of energy of the erythrocytes.

Makrosymprotite

Patient: P., geb. 1986
Diagnose: Hohes Fieber über mehrere Wochen

Macrosymprotits

Patient: P., born 1986
Diagnosis: High fever for several weeks

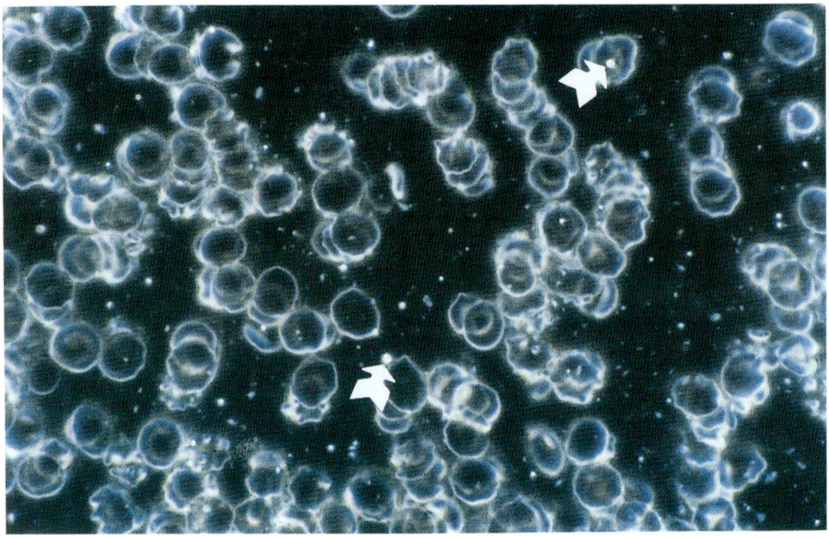

Aufnahme von: 12/1988 – Photo taken: 12/1988

Bewertung: ➽ Makrosymprotite im Plasma – Symbiosestörung; hohe Aktivität der Symbionten im Plasma – akute Infektion; verformte Erythrozyten – endobiontische Belastung (1 h nach Blutentnahme).

Evaluation: ➽ Macrosymprotits in the plasma – disturbance of symbiosis; high activity of the symbionts in the plasma – acute infection; deformed erythrocytes – endobiontic burden (one hour after taking of blood sample).

Freie Chondrite

Patientin: E., geb. 1979
Diagnose: Rez. Cystitis, Rhinitis allergica, Pollenallergie

Free chondrits

Patient (female): E., born 1979
Diagnosis: Recurring cystitis, rhinitis allergica, pollen allergy

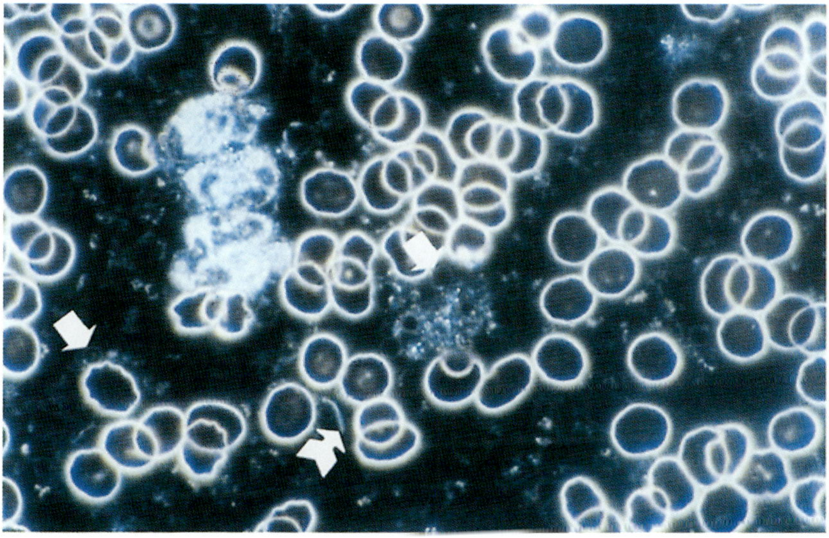

Aufnahme von: 7/1990 – Photo taken: 7/1990

Bewertung: Freier Chondrit im Plasma (➽); Agglutination von mehreren Granulozyten, Befall der Granulozyten durch sporoide Symprotite – zelluläre Abwehr geschwächt; mehrere Kolloidthecite im Plasma (➡) – Abwehrbereitschaft des symbiontischen Systems.

Evaluation: Free chondrit in the plasma (➽) agglutination of several granulocytes, infestation of the granulocytes by sporoid symprotits – weakened cellular defence; several colloid-thecits in the plasma (➡) – defence readiness of the symbiontic system.

Mychit

Patientin:	D., geb. 1936
Diagnose:	Durchblutungsstörungen, Hämorrhoiden

Mychit

Patient (female):	D., born 1936
Diagnosis:	Disturbances of blood supply, haemorrhoids

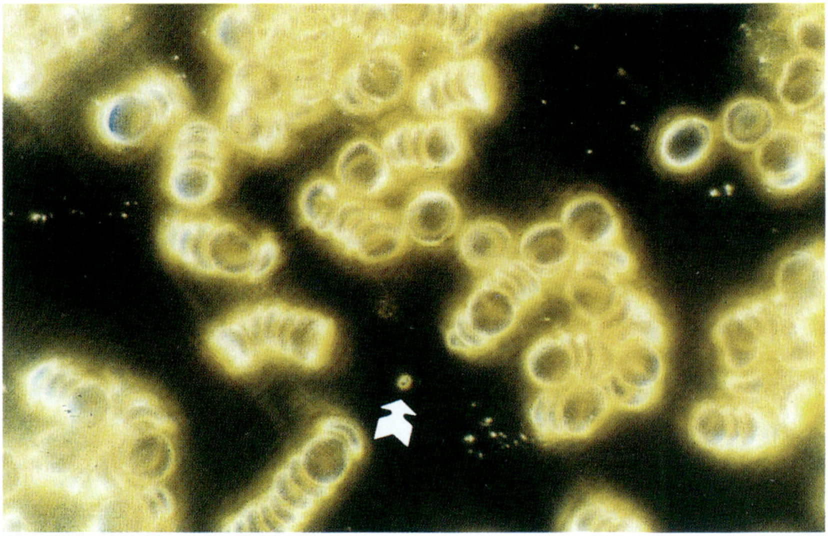

Aufnahme von: 8/1992 – Photo taken: 8/1992

Bewertung: ➽ Mychit mit wandständigem Kern – pathogene Form des Endobionten; Agglutination der Erythrozyten – Endobiose.

Evaluation: ➽ Mychit with parietal nucleus – pathogenic form from the endobiont; agglutination of the erythrocytes – endobiosis.

Thecite

Patient: P., geb. 1908
Diagnose: Blasen-Ca, Durchblutungsstörungen in beiden Beinen, Gastritis, Colitis ulcerosa, Angina pectoris

Thecits

Patient: P., born 1908
Diagnosis: Carcinoma of the bladder, disturbances of blood supply in both legs, gastritis, ulcerous colitis, angina pectoris

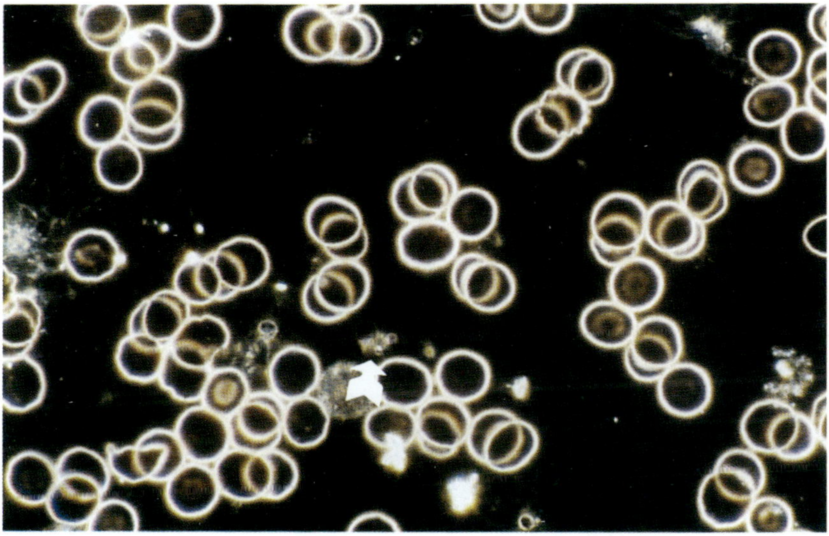

Aufnahme von: 1/1993 – Photo taken: 1/1993

Bewertung: ➽ Konglomerat eines Thrombozyten mit 2 Theciten; Erythrozyten endobiontisch verformt (1 h nach Blutentnahme).

Evaluation: ➽ Conglomeration of a thrombocyte with 2 thecits; erythrocytes with endobiontic deformation (one hour after taking of blood sample).

Thrombozyten

Patient: R., geb. 1947
Diagnose: Sinusitis frontalis, Durchblutungsstörungen

Thrombocytes

Patient: R., born 1947
Diagnosis: Sinusitis frontalis, disturbances of blood supply

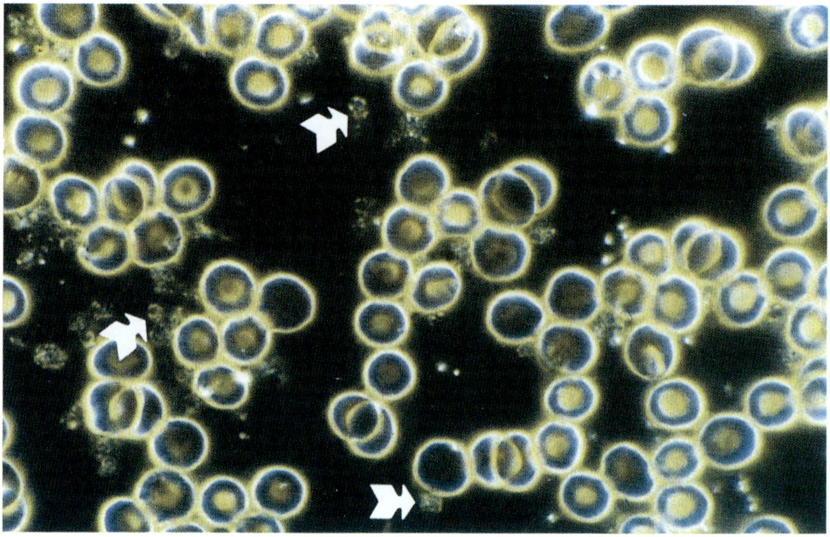

Aufnahme von: 12/1992 – Photo taken: 12/1992

Bewertung: ➽ Zahlreiche Thrombozyten im Plasma; Erythrozyten endobiontisch belastet.

Evaluation: ➽ Numerous thrombocytes in the plasma; erythrocytes with endobiontic burden.

Patientin: G., geb. 1925
Diagnose: Herzinfarkt (1972), Durchblutungsstörungen

Patient (female): G., born 1925
Diagnosis: Cardiac infarction (1972), disturbances of blood supply

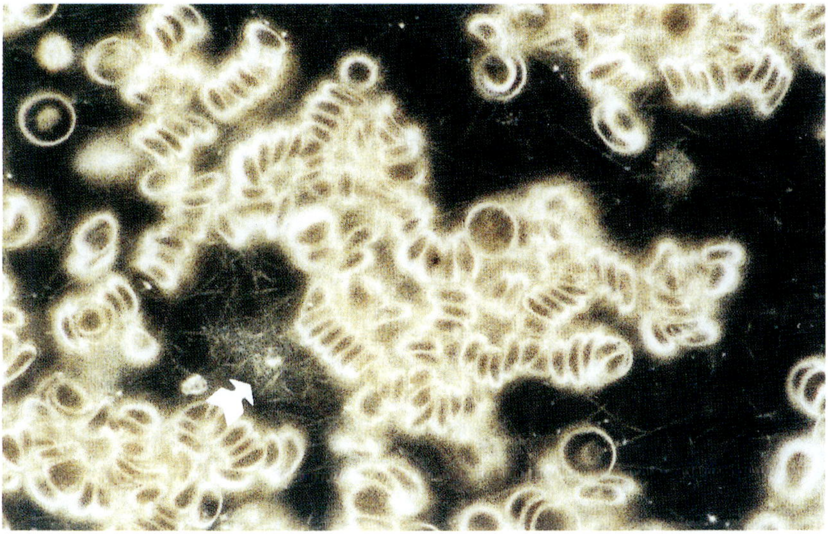

Aufnahme von: 9/1992 – Photo taken: 9/1992

Bewertung: ➽ Zusammengeballte Thrombozyten mit Filiten, Agglutination der Erythrozyten – Endobiose.

Evaluation: ➽ Accumulated thrombocytes with filits, agglutination of the erythrocytes – endobiosis.

Kolloidthecite

Patientin: E., geb. 1979
Diagnose: Rez. Cystitis, Rhinitis allergica, Pollenallergie

Colloid-thecits

Patient (female): E., born 1979
Diagnosis: Recurring cystitis, rhinitis allergica, pollen allergy

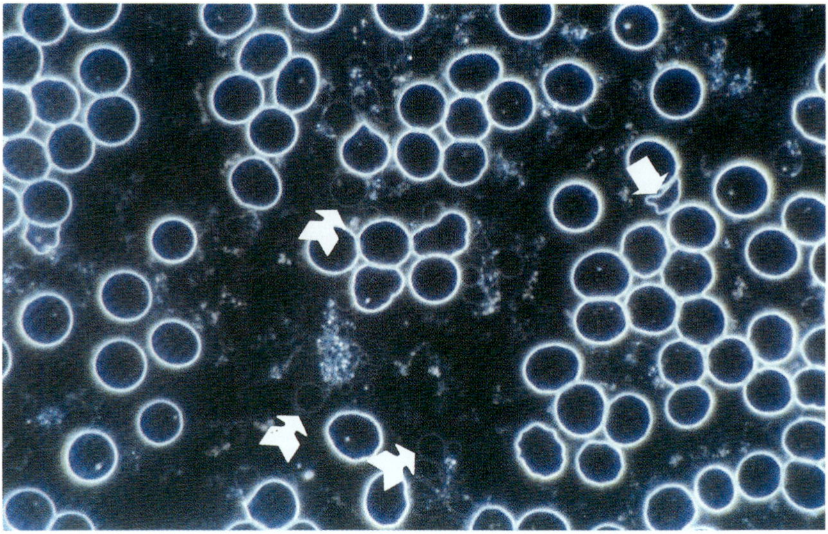

Aufnahme von: 7/1990 – Photo taken: 7/1990

Bewertung: ➽ Zahlreiche Kolloidthecite im Plasma – Abwehrbereitschaft; ➡ rechts oben sich verkleinernder Erythrozyt mit schlauchförmiger Ausstülpung (Bildung eines Bakterienstäbchens) – endobiontische Belastung; Erythrozytenmembranen stark lumineszierend – nach Prigge Energieschwäche der E.

Evaluation: ➽ Numerous colloid-thecits in the plasma – defence readiness; ➡ on top to the right, erythrocyte reducing in size with tubular protrusion (formation of a bacterial rod) – endobiontic burden; membranes of the erythrocytes with strong luminescence – according to Prigge weakness of energy of the erythrocytes.

Diökothecite

Patient: F., geb. 1966
Diagnose: Apoplex

Dioeko-thecits

Patient: F., born 1966
Diagnosis: Apoplexia

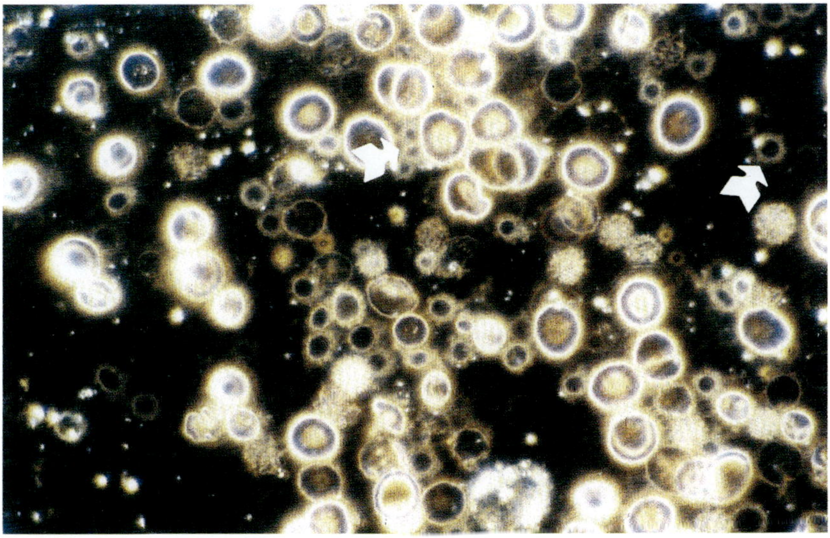

Aufnahme von: 8/1992 – Photo taken: 8/1992

Bewertung: ➽ Zahlreiche Diökothecite im Plasma – Abwehrbereitschaft; Erythrozyten stark endobiontisch belastet – schweres Krankheitsbild.

Evaluation: ➽ Numerous dioeko-thecits in the plasma – defence readiness; erythrocytes with strong endobiontic burden – severe pathological picture.

Patientin: R., geb. 1945
Diagnose: Osteomyelosklerose

Patient (female): R., born 1945
Diagnosis: Osteomyelosclerosis

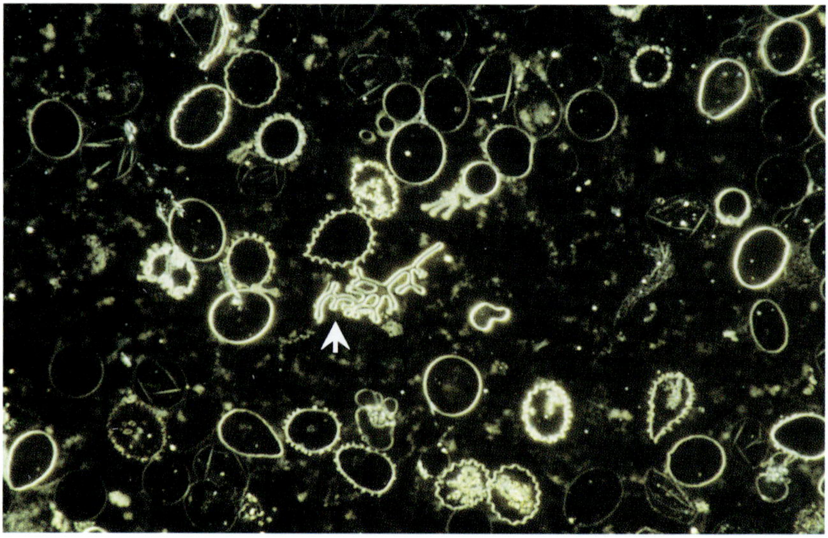

Aufnahme von: 2/1999 – Photo taken: 2/1999

Bewertung: In der Mitte Konglomerat von teilweise verzweigten Bakterienstäbchen (Leptotrichia buccalis) – starke Endobiose; Erythrozyten endobiontisch belastet, Anisozytose – Anämie (1 h nach Blutentnahme).

Evaluation: In the centre bacterial rod (Leptotrichia buccalis) – strong endobiosis; erythrocytes with endobiontic burden, anisocytosis – anemia (one hour after blood sample).

Patientin: R., geb. 1945
Diagnose: Osteomyelosklerose

Patient (female): R., born 1945
Diagnosis: Osteomyelosclerosis

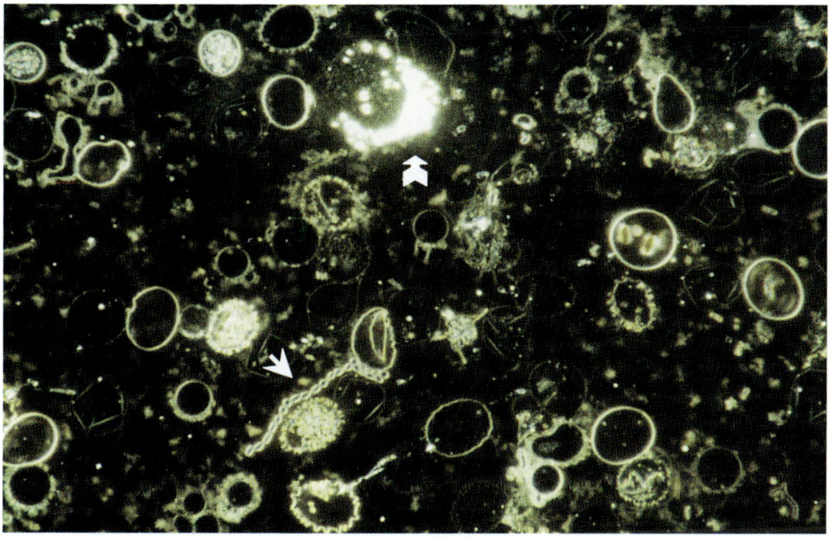

Aufnahme von: 2/1999 – Photo taken: 2/1999

Bewertung: ➘ In der Mitte Mychitkette der Leptotrichia buccalis – starke Endobiose;
⮝ oben zerfallender Granulozyt – geschwächte zelluläre Abwehr (1 h nach Blutentnahme).

Evaluation: ➘ In the centre chain of mychites (Leptotrichia buccalis) – strong endobiosis;
⮝ above granulocyte in state of degradation – weakened cellular defence (one hour after blood sample).

Patient: Sch., geb. 1945
Diagnose: Angina pectoris

Patient: Sch., born 1945
Diagnosis: Angina pectoris

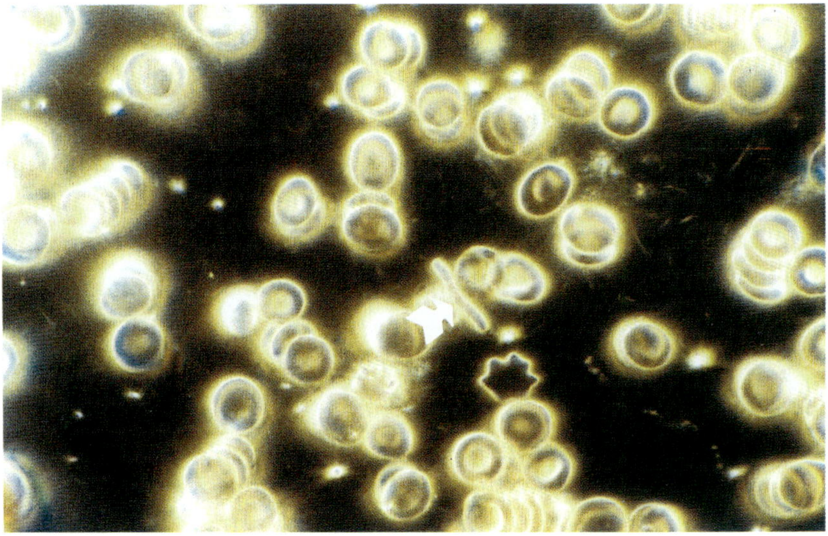

Aufnahme von: 12/1993 – Photo taken: 12/1993

Bewertung: ➽ In der Bildmitte Bakterienstäbchen (Leptotrichia buccalis), Erythrozyten endobiontisch belastet.

Evaluation: ➽ In the cetre bacterial rod (Leptotrichia buccalis), erythrocytes with endobiontic burden.

Symplasten, sklerotische Formen und kristallähnliche Strukturen

Patientin: L., geb. 1937
Diagnose: Rheumatische Beschwerden, CWS-Syndrom, Oberbauch-Syndrom

Symplasts, sclerotic forms and crystal-like structures

Patient (female): L., born 1937
Diagnosis: Rheumatic troubles, CVS-syndrome, upper abdomen syndrome

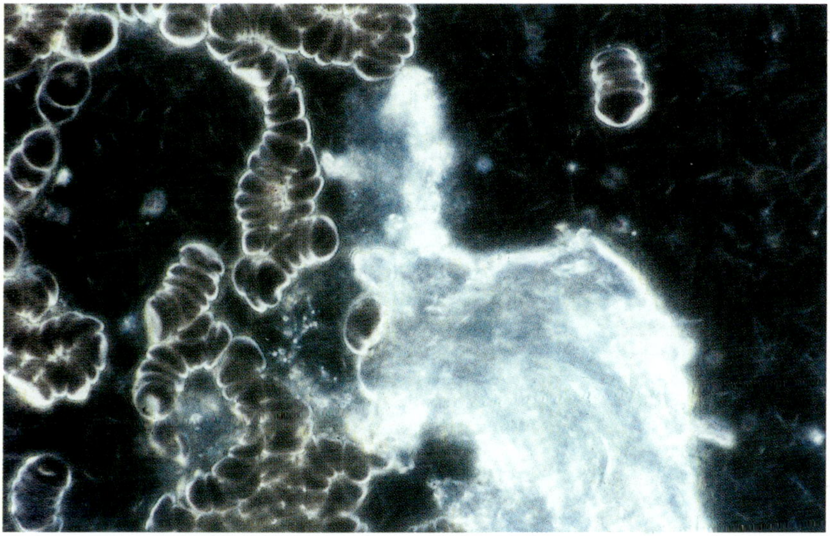

Aufnahme von: 12/1988 – Photo taken: 12/1988

Bewertung: „Mucor-Symplast", starke Geldrollenbildung, im Plasma leichte Filitbildung – Endobiose.

Evaluation: „Mucor symplast", strong coin roll formation, in the plasma slight filit formation – endobiosis.

Patient: W., geb. 1956, † 1991
Diagnose: Aids

Patient: W., born 1956, † 1991
Diagnosis: Aids

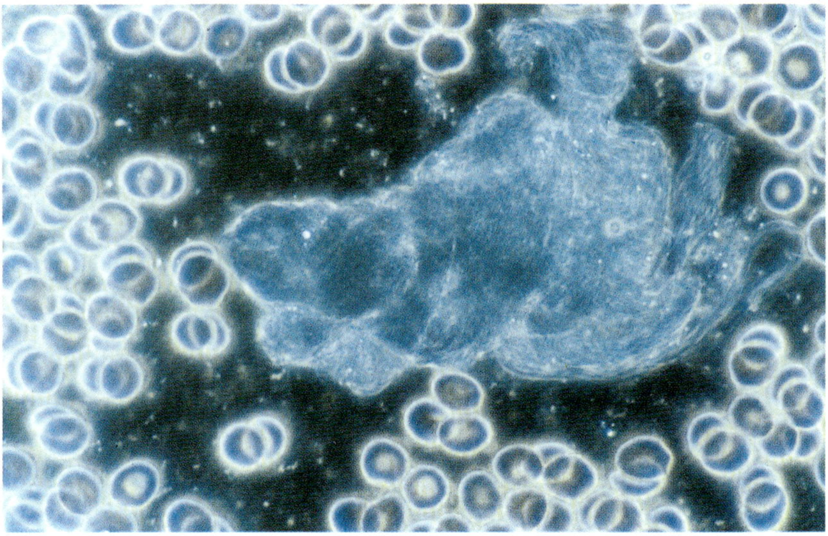

Aufnahme von: 2/1990 – Photo taken: 2/1990

Bewertung: Dunkler Symplast – Konglomerat von parasitären Formen des Aspergillus niger-Zyklus; erhöhte Lumineszenz der Erythrozytenmembranen; Erythrozyten endobiontisch belastet.

Evaluation: Dark symplast – conglomeration of parasitic forms of the Aspergillus niger cyclodes; increased luminescence of the erythrocyte membranes; erythrocytes with endobiontic burden.

Patientin: P., geb. 1984
Diagnose: Neurodermitis, Alopezie

Patient (female): P., born 1984
Diagnosis: Neurodermitis, alopecia

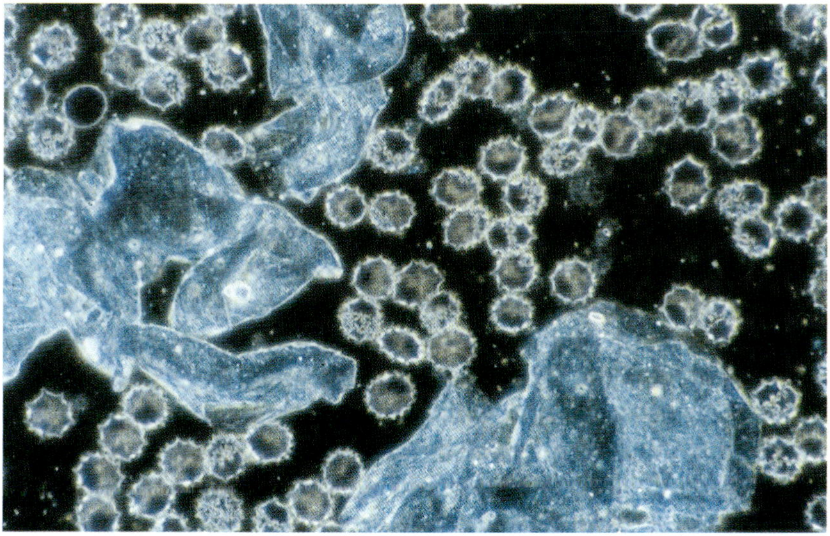

Aufnahme von: 10/1990 – Photo taken: 10/1990

Bewertung: Mehrere große dunkle Symplasten – Belastung mit parasitären Formen der Aspergillus niger-Zyklode; Erythrozyten endobiontisch befallen (Stechapfelformen).

Evaluation: Several big, dark symplasts - burdening with parasitic forms of the Aspergillus niger cyclode; erythrocytes with endobiontic infestation (thorn-apple-forms).

Patientin: G., geb. 1916
Diagnose: Mamma-Ca rechts, Durchblutungsstörungen in beiden Augen

Patient (female): G., born 1916
Diagnosis: Cancer of the right breast, disturbances of blood supply in both eyes

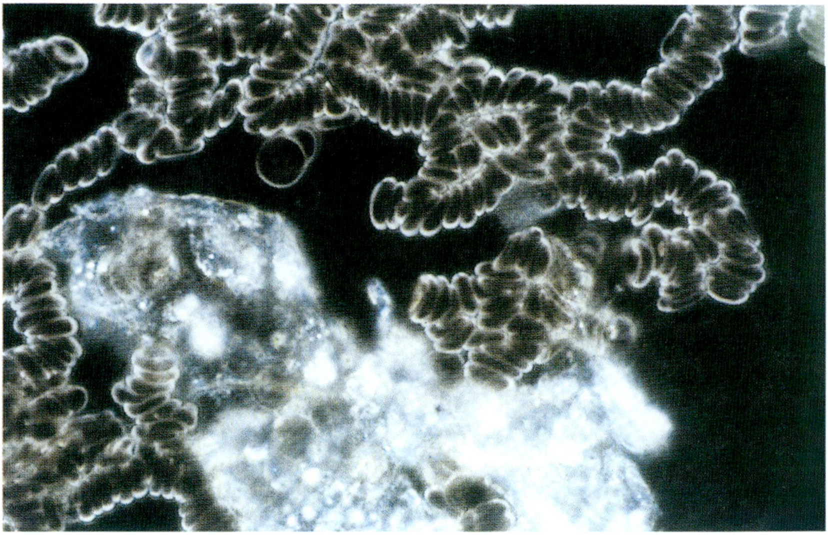

Aufnahme von: 4/1990 – Photo taken: 4/1990

Bewertung: Symplast mit sporoiden Symprotiten – Nierenbelastung; starke Geldrollenbildung – Durchblutungsstörungen, Stauungen; Plasma ohne Symbionten – keine symbiontische Abwehr, Blockade.

Evaluation: Symplast with sporoid symprotits – kidney stress; strong coin roll formation – disturbances of blood supply; congestions; plasma without symbionts – no symbiontic defence, blockage.

Patient:	Sch., geb. 1944
Diagnose:	CWS-Syndrom
Patient:	Sch., born 1944
Diagnosis:	CVS-syndrome

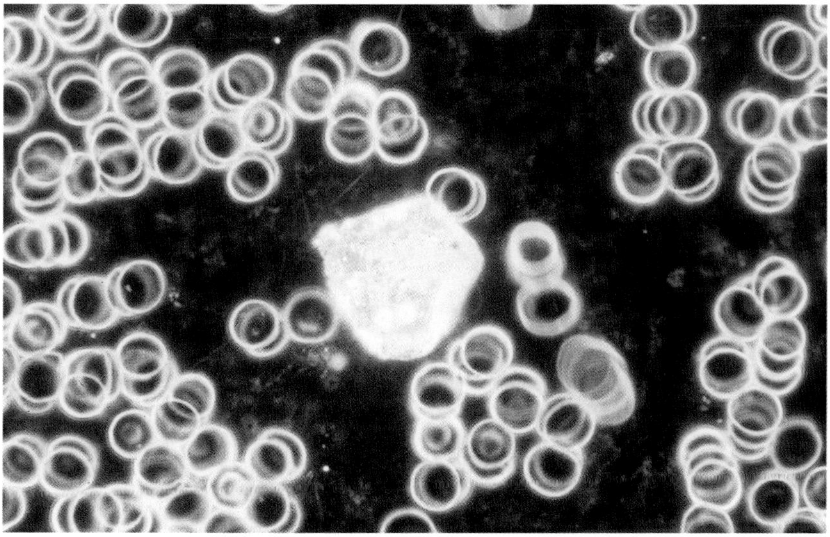

Aufnahme von: 2/1990 – Photo taken: 2/1990

Bewertung: Symplast, durch Agglutination von Leukozyten entstanden; leichte Geldrollenbildung – leichte Endobiose.

Evaluation: Symplast, developed from agglutination of leucocytes; slight coin roll formation, slight endobiosis.

Patientin:	R., geb. 1935
Diagnose:	Oberbauchsyndrom, Durchfälle, Colon-Divertikel, Pilzbefall im Darm (Candida albicans)

Patient (female):	R., born 1935
Diagnosis:	Upper abdomen syndrome, diarrheas, diverticulum of the colon, fungal infestation of the intestine (Candida albicans)

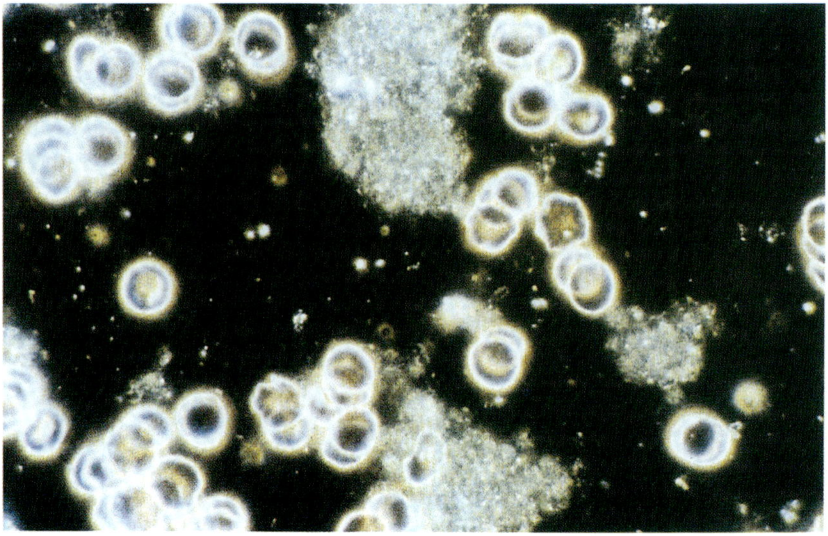

Aufnahme von: 2/1992 – Photo taken: 2/1992

Bewertung: Mehrere sich auflösende Symplasten, Erythrozyten endobiontisch belastet.

Evaluation: Several symplasts in states of degradation, erythrocytes with endobiontic burden.

Patient: V., geb. 1936
Diagnose: Arteriosklerose der Becken- und der Oberschenkelarterie, Leber- und Nierenbelastung, LWS-Syndrom

Patient: V., born 1936
Diagnosis: Arteriosclerosis of the artery of the pelvis and the femur, liver and kidney stress, lumbar-vertebral syndrome

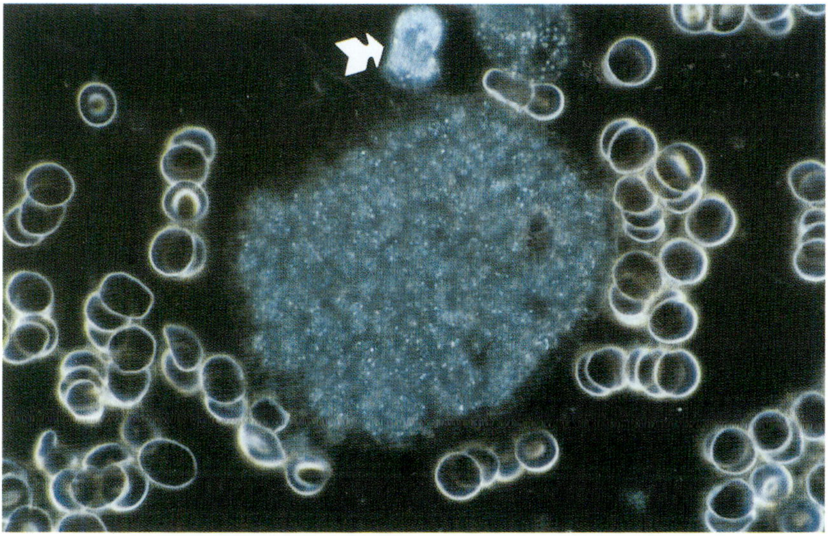

Aufnahme von: 5/1989 – Photo taken: 5/1989

Bewertung: Sich auflösender grüner Symplast – Nierenbelastung, einzelne zitronenförmige Erythrozyten – leichte Leberbelastung; oberhalb des Symplasten Granulozyt ➽.

Evaluation: Green symplast in state of degradation – kidney stress; occasional lemon-shaped erythrocytes – slight liver stress, above the symplast – granulozyte ➽.

Patient: K., geb. 1938
Diagnose: Thrombophlebitis, Ulcus cruris an beiden Beinen

Patient: K., born 1938
Diagnosis: Thrombophlebitis, varicose ulcer on both legs

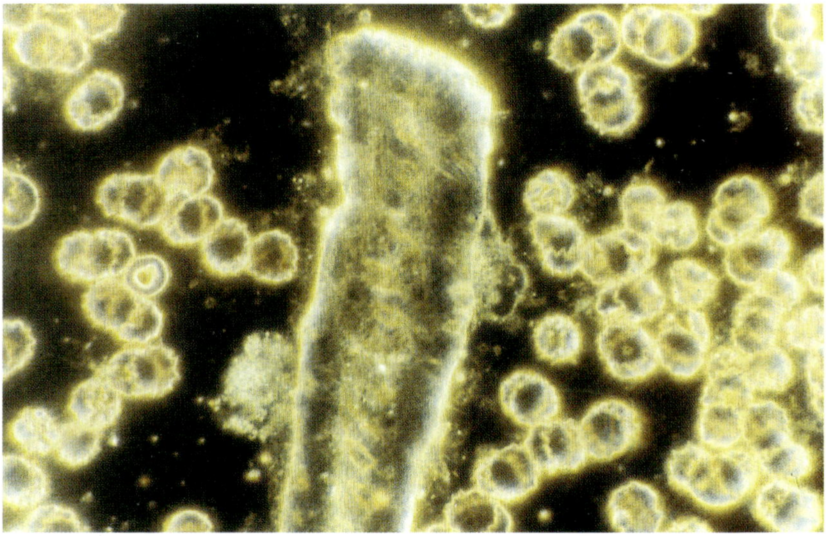

Aufnahme von: 7/1992 – Photo taken: 7/1992

Bewertung: „Aspergillus-Symplast", der von 2 Leukozyten attackiert wird; Endobiose der Erythrozyten (1 h nach Blutabnahme).

Evaluation: „Aspergillus-symplast" which is attacked by two leucocytes; endobiosis of the erythrocytes (one hour after taking blood sample).

Patientin: R., geb. 1945
Diagnose: Osteomyelosklerose

Patient (female): R., born 1945
Diagnosis: Osteomyelosclerosis

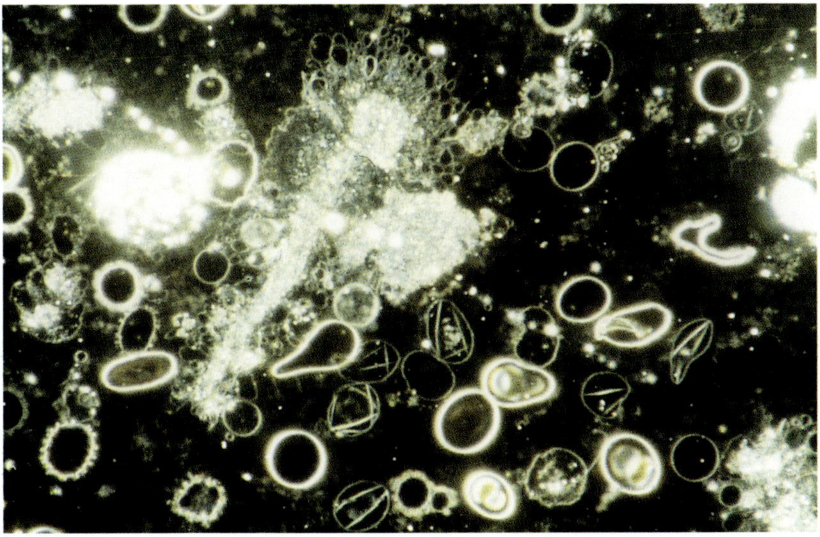

Aufnahme von: 2/1999 – Photo taken: 2/1999

Bewertung: In der Mitte durch Zusammenballung von Leukozyten entstehender Symplast – starke endobiontische Belastung der Leukozyten; birnenförmige Erythrozyten – Milzbelastung; starke endobiontische Belastung der Erythrozyten (1 h nach Blutentnahme).

Evaluation: In the centre symplast from leucocytes – strong endobiontic burden of leucocytes; pear-shaped erythrocytes – spleen stress; erythrocytes with strong endobiontic burden (one hour after blood sample).

Patientin: B., geb. 1941
Diagnose: Totale Virus-Bakterien-Intoxikation, Nierenbelastung (OP Zyste Niere rechts)

Patient (female): B., born 1941
Diagnosis: Total intoxication with viruses and bacteria, kidney stress (operation right kidney with cyst removal)

Aufnahme 1 – Photo 1

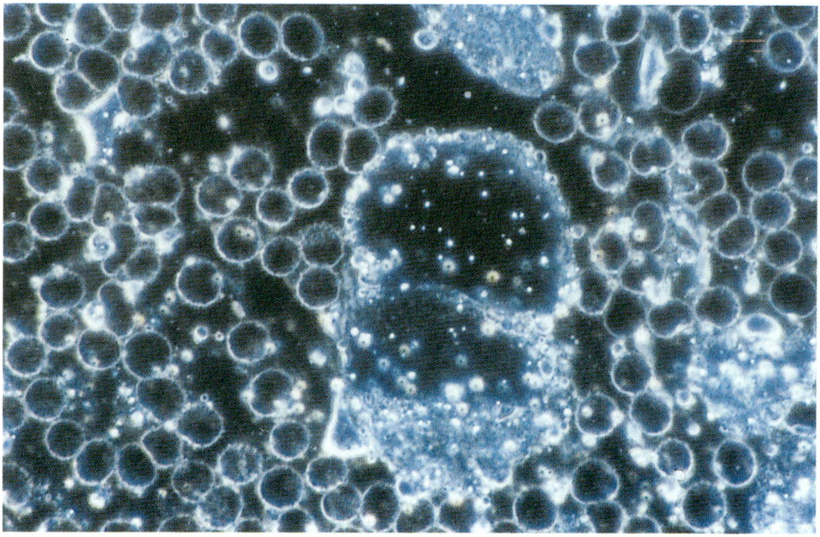

Aufnahme von: 12/1988 – Photo taken: 12/1988

Bewertung: Dunkler Sklerosymplast mit sporoiden Symprotiten; Erythrozyten mit Randbesatz – Endobiose.

Evaluation: Dark sclerosymplast with sporoid symprotit; erythrocytes with marginal edgings – endobiosis.

Aufnahme 2 – Photo 2

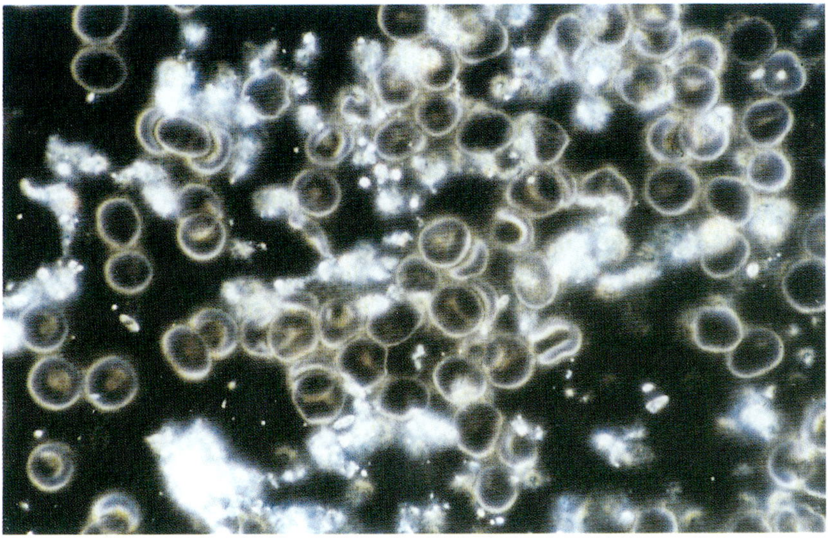

Aufnahme von: 12/1988 – Photo taken: 12/1988

Bewertung: Zusammengeballte sporoide Symprotite – Nierenbelastung.

Evaluation: Conglomeration of sporoid symprotits – kidney stress.

Patientin: B., geb. 1911
Diagnose: Pankreas-Ca

Patient (female): B., born 1911
Diagnosis: Carcinoma of the pancreas

Aufnahme 1 – Photo 1

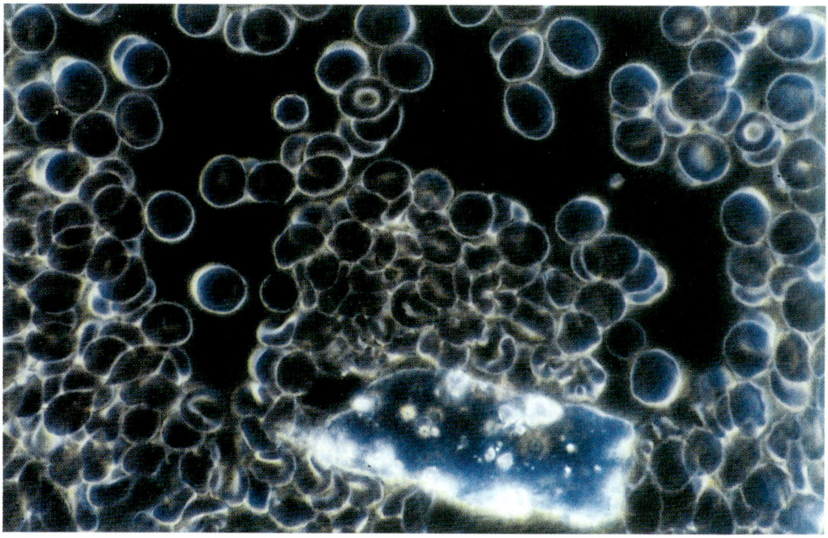

Aufnahme von: 2/1989 – Photo taken: 2/1989

Bewertung: Dunkler Sklerosymplast am unteren Bildrand; Erythrozyten endobiontisch belastet, starke Agglutination, zitronenförmige E. – Leberbelastung.

Evaluation: Dark sclerosymplast at the lower edge of picture; erythrocytes with endobiontic burden, strong agglutination, lemon-shaped erythrocytes – liver burden.

Patientin: B., geb. 1911
Diagnose: Pankreas-Ca

Patient (female): B., born 1911
Diagnosis: Carcinoma of the pancreas

Aufnahme 2 – Photo 2

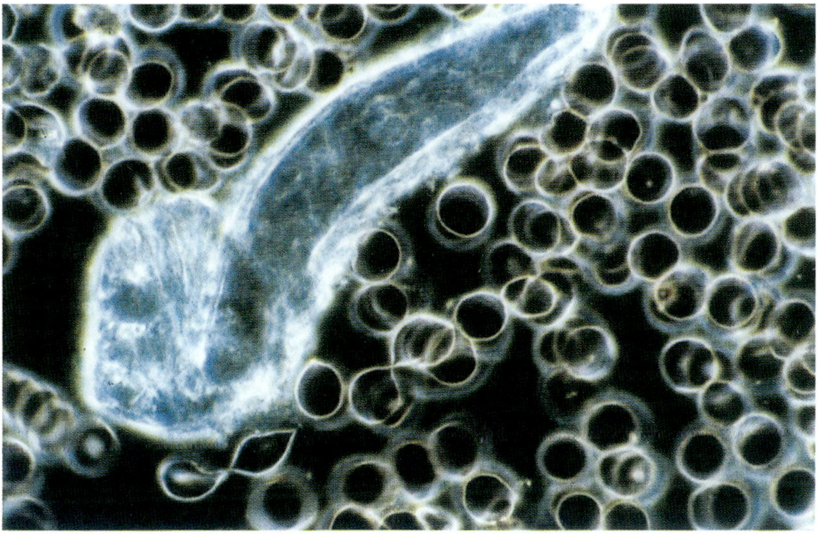

Aufnahme von: 2/1989 – Photo taken: 2/1989

Bewertung: „Aspergillus-Symplast"; zitronenförmige Erythrozyten – Leberbelastung.

Evaluation: „Aspergillus-symplast"; lemon-shaped erythrocytes – liver burden.

Patientin: B., geb. 1911
Diagnose: Pankreas-Ca

Patient (female): B., born 1911
Diagnosis: Carcinoma of the pancreas

Aufnahme 3 – Photo 3

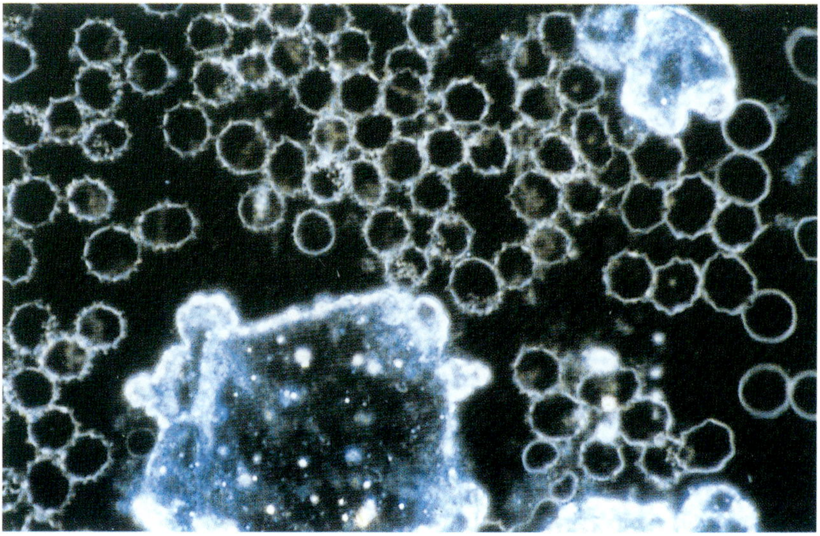

Aufnahme von: 2/1989 – Photo taken: 2/1989

Bewertung: Dunkle Sklerosymplasten; Erythrozyten mit Randbesatz – starke Endobiose, schweres Krankheitsbild.

Evaluation: Dark sclerosymplasts; erythrocytes with marginal edgings – strong endobiosis, severe pathogenic symptom.

Patient: K., geb. 1943
Diagnose: Cholezystitis

Patient: K., geb. 1943
Diagnosis: Cholecystitis

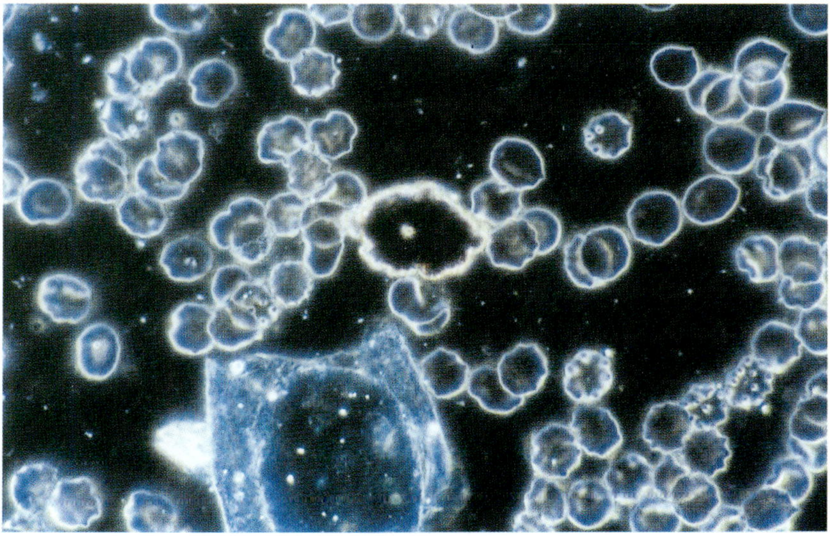

Aufnahme von: 2/1989 – Photo taken: 2/1989

Bewertung: In der Bildmitte brauner Sklerosymplast – Oberbauchbelastung; am unteren Bildrand dunkler „kristalliner Symplast"; Erythrozyten endobiontisch belastet, mit Vakuolen und Randzacken – Endobiose, vereinzelt zitronenförmige E. – Leberbelastung.

Evaluation: In the centre of the picture brown sclerosymplast – upper abdomen stress; at the lower edge of picture dark „crystalline symplast", erythrocytes with endobiontic burden, with vacuoles and marginal points – endobiosis, occasional lemon-shaped erythrocytes – liver burden.

Patient: H., geb. 1932
Diagnose: Erkrankung der Peyerschen Plaques (Dünndarm)

Patient: H., born 1932
Diagnosis: Disease of Peyer's Patches (small intestine)

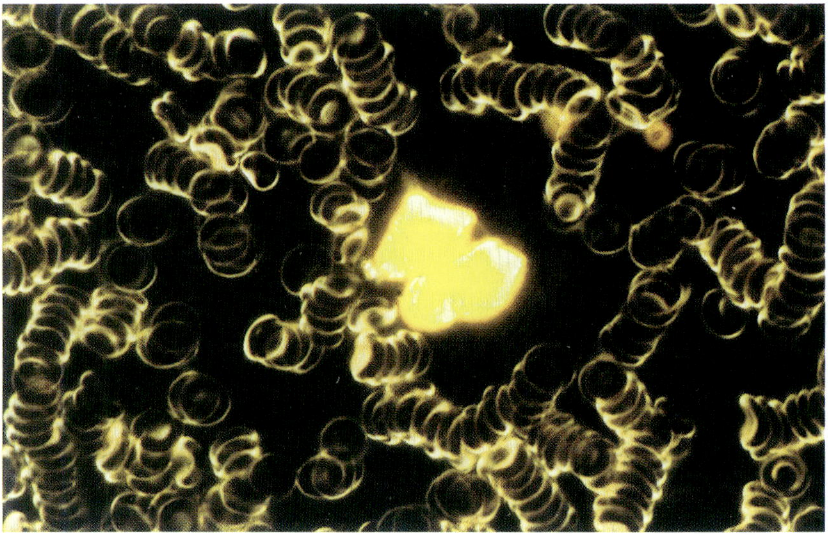

Aufnahme von: 8/1992 – Photo taken: 8/1992

Bewertung: Zitronengelbe symplastähnliche Struktur – Hinweis auf Oberbauch; leicht gebogene Geldrollen – nach Prigge Hinweis auf Darmbelastung.

Evaluation: Lemon yellow symplast-like structure – indication to upper abdomen; slightly curved coin rolls – according to Prigge indication to intestinal stress.

Patient: Z., geb. 1930
Diagnose: Chronische Pankreatitis

Patient: Z., born 1930
Diagnosis: Chronic pancreatitis

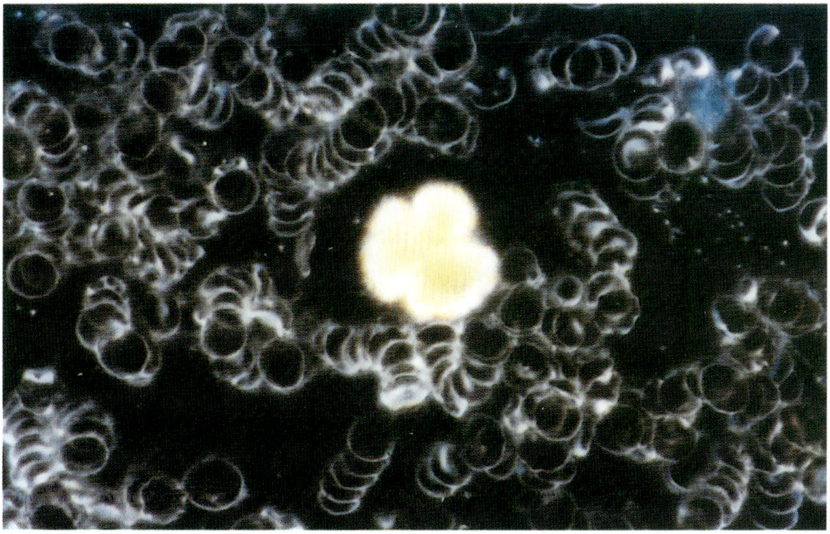

Aufnahme von: 12/1988 – Photo taken: 12/1988

Bewertung: Gelber Sklerosymplast – Hinweis auf Oberbauch, starke Aggregation der Erythrozyten – Stauungen.

Evaluation: Yellow sclerosymplast – indication to upper abdomen, strong aggregation of erythrocytes – congestions.

Patientin: K., geb. 1969
Diagnose: Chronische Cystitis, Nierenbelastung, chronische Sinusitis (Fehldiagnose MS)

Patient (female): K., born 1969
Diagnosis: Chronic cystitis, kidney stress, chronic sinusitis (false diagnosis of multiple sclerosis)

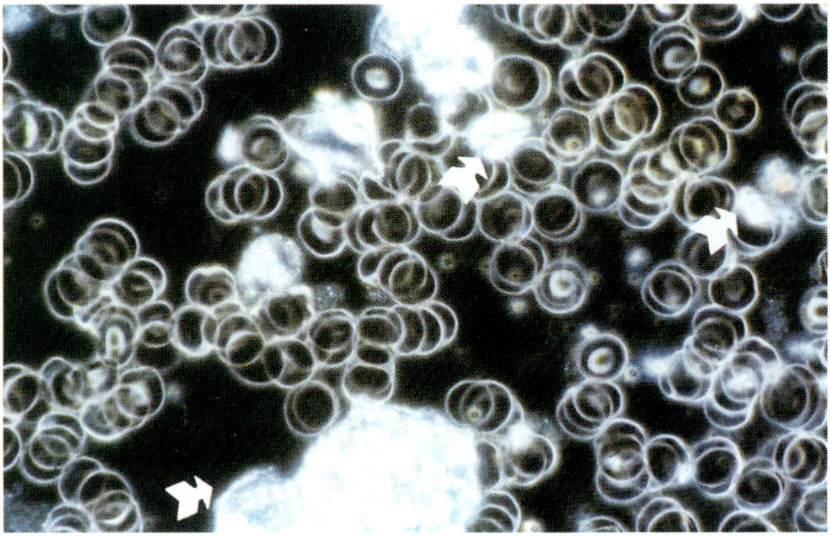

Aufnahme von: 4/1990 – Photo taken: 4/1990

Bewertung: ➽ Weißes symplastähnliches Gebilde und Kristalle – Hinweis auf Nierenbelastung.

Evaluation: ➽ White symplast-like formation and crystals – indication to kidney stress.

Patientin: A., geb. 1946
Diagnose: Roemheld, uratische Diathese mit „Aspergillus-Beteiligung"

Patient (female): A., born 1946
Diagnosis: Roemheld, uratic diathesis with „Aspergillus implication"

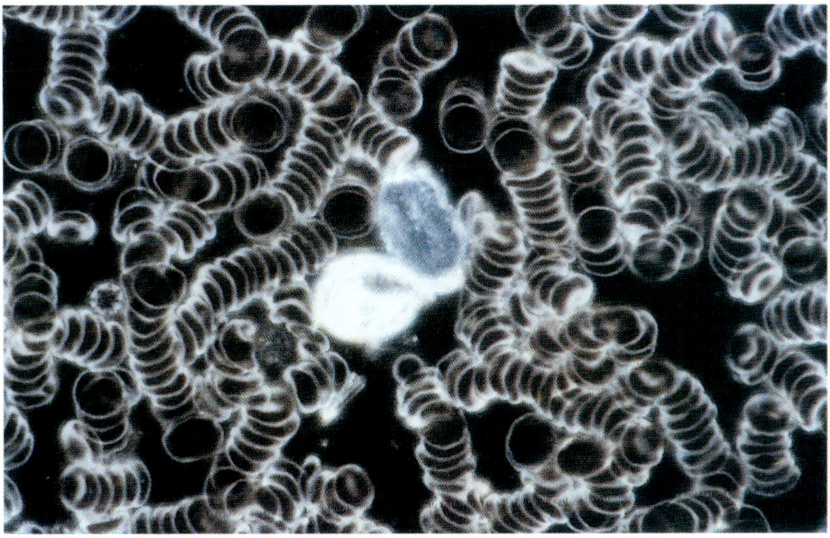

Aufnahme von: 10/1990 – Photo taken: 10/1990

Bewertung: Symplastform – Hinweis auf Nierenbelastung; gebogene Geldrollen nach Prigge (1990) Hinweis auf Darmbelastung.

Evaluation: Symplast formation – indication to kidney stress; curved coin rolls – according to Prigge (1990) indication to intestinal stress.

Patient: N., geb. 1955
Diagnose: Belastung der rechten Niere

Patient: N., born 1955
Diagnosis: Stress of right kidney

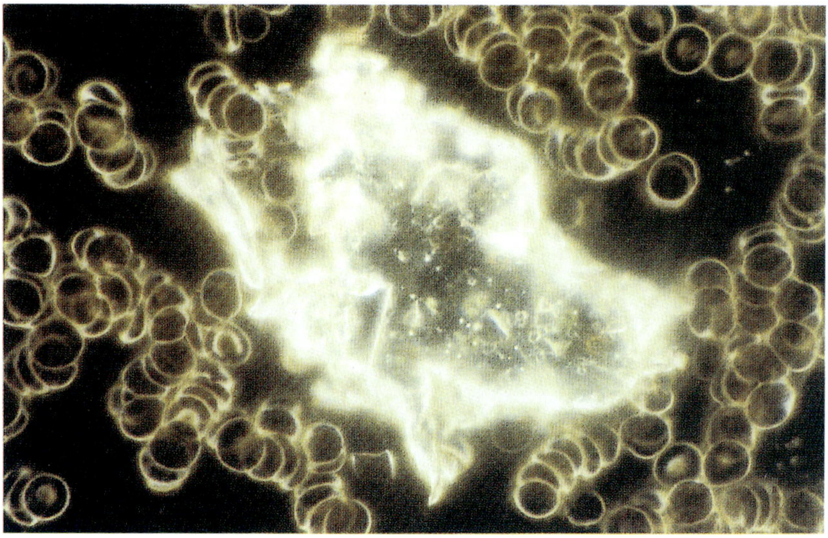

Aufnahme von: 6/1992 – Photo taken: 6/1992

Bewertung: Grüner Sklerosymplast – Nierenbelastung; Agglutination der Erythrozyten – Endobiose.

Evaluation: Green sclerosymplast – kidney stress: agglutination of erythrocytes – endobiosis.

Patientin: T., geb. 1937
Diagnose: Cystitis, chronische Gastritis

Patient (female): T., born 1937
Diagnosis: Cystitis, chronic gastritis

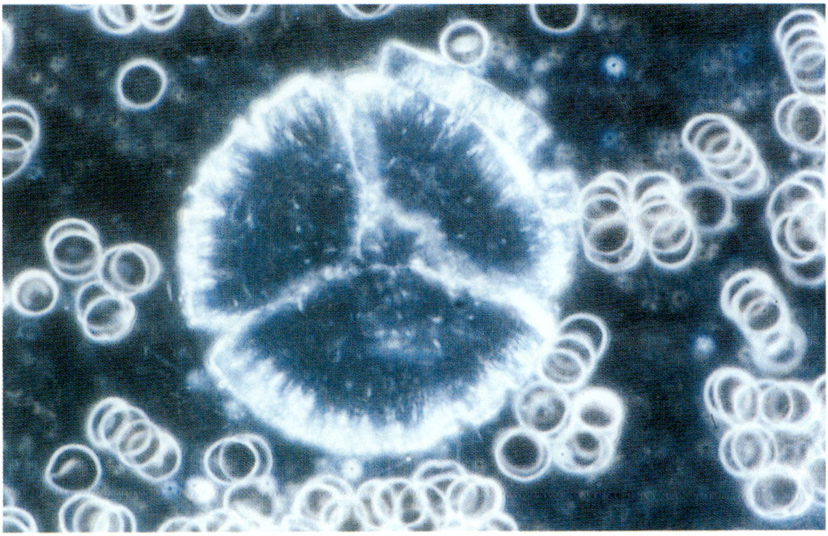

Aufnahme von: 2/1990 – Photo taken: 2/1990

Bewertung: Scheibenförmiger segmentierter Sklerosymplast – Hinweis auf Urogenitaltrakt (Blase).

Evaluation: Disc-shaped segmented sclerosymplast – indication to urogenital tract (bladder).

Patientin: M., geb. 1942
Diagnose: Morbus Bechterew, akute Cystitis

Patient (female): M., born 1942
Diagnosis: Morbus Bechterew, acute cystitis

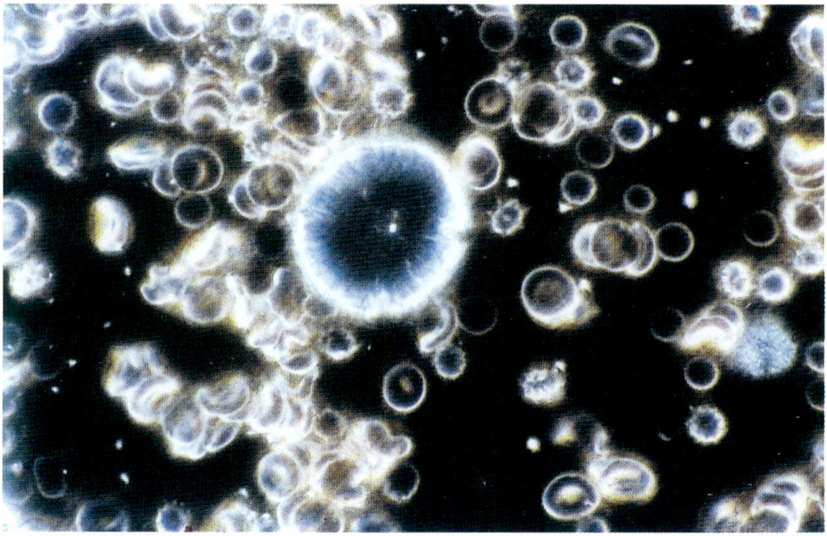

Aufnahme von: 12/1988 – Photo taken: 12/1988

Bewertung: Scheibenförmiger Sklerosymplast – Hinweis auf Urogenitaltrakt (Blase); endobiontische Belastung der Erythrozyten.

Evaluation: Disc-shaped sclerosymplast – indication to urogenital tract (bladder); endobiotic burden of erythrocytes.

Patientin:	M., geb. 1968
Diagnose:	Chronische Cystitis

Patient (female):	M., born 1968
Diagnosis:	Chronic cystitis

Aufnahme 1 – Photo 1

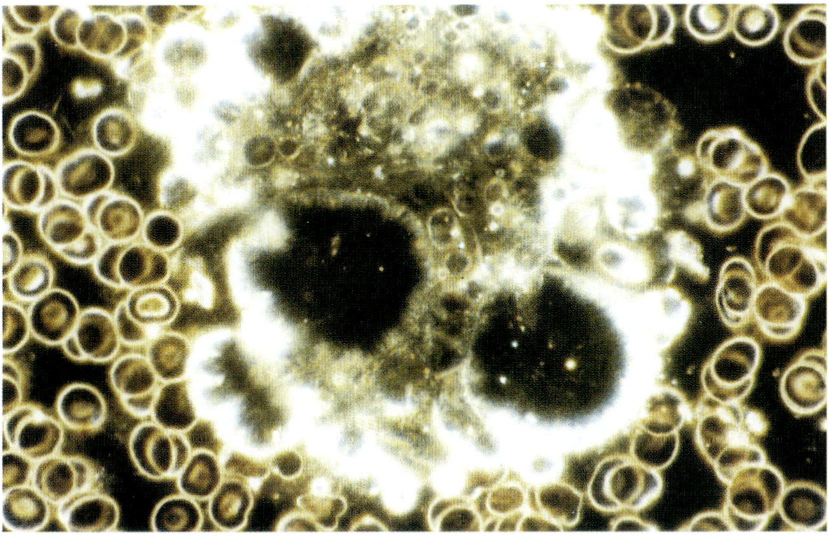

Aufnahme von: 11/1992 – Photo taken: 11/1992

B e w e r t u n g: Riesiges sklerotisches Gebilde mit mehreren scheibenförmigen Sklero-symplasten – Hinweis auf Urogenitaltrakt (Blase).

E v a l u a t i o n: Huge sclerotic formation with several disc-shaped sclerosymplasts – indication to urogenitel tract (bladder).

Patientin: M., geb. 1968
Diagnose: Chronische Cystitis

Patient (female): M., born 1968
Diagnosis: Chronic cystitis

Aufnahme 2 – Photo 2

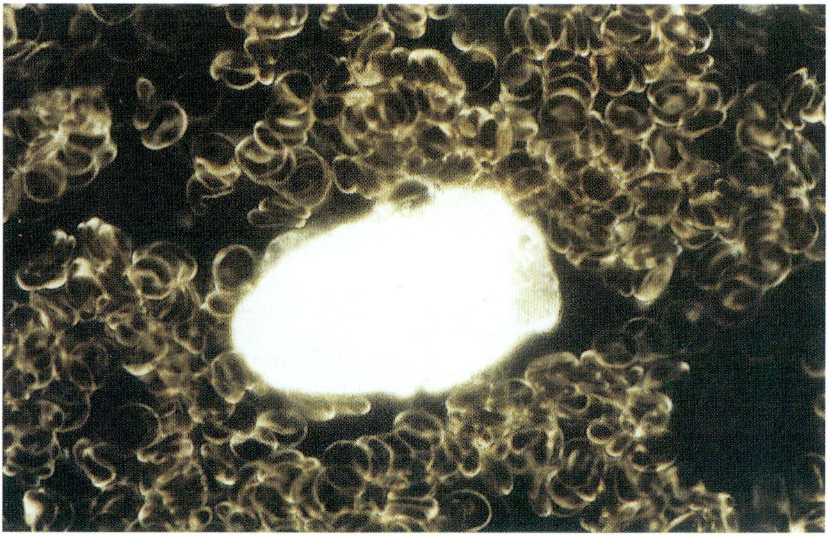

Aufnahme von: 11/1992 – Photo taken: 11/1992

Bewertung: Weißes symplastähnliches Gebilde – Beteiligung der Nieren.

Evaluation: Huge sclerotic formation with several disc-shaped sclerosymplasts.

Patientin: N., geb. 1987
Diagnose: Akute lymphatische Leukämie

Patient (female): N., born 1987
Diagnosis: Acute lymphatic leukaemia

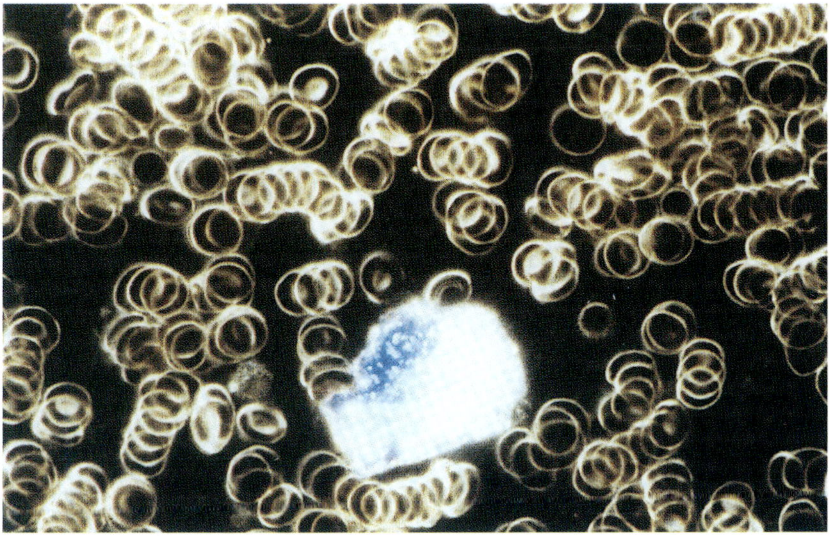

Aufnahme von: 9/1992 – Photo taken: 9/1992

Bewertung: Kornblumenblauer Symplast – Hinweis auf Schilddrüse; Agglutination der Erythrozyten – Endobiose,- Symbiontenaktivität gering – schwache symbiontische Abwehr

Evaluation: Cornflower blue symplast – indication to thyroid gland; agglutination of erythrocytes – endobiosis; minor symbiontic activity – weak symbiontic defence.

Patientin: E., geb. 1952
Diagnose: Ulcus ventriculi, Ulcus duodeni, chronische Sinusitis, Stauungen im linken Lenden-Unterbauch-Bereich

Patient (female): E., born 1952
Diagnosis: Round ulcer, duodenal ulcer, chronic sinusitis, congestions in the area of the left loin and lower abdomen

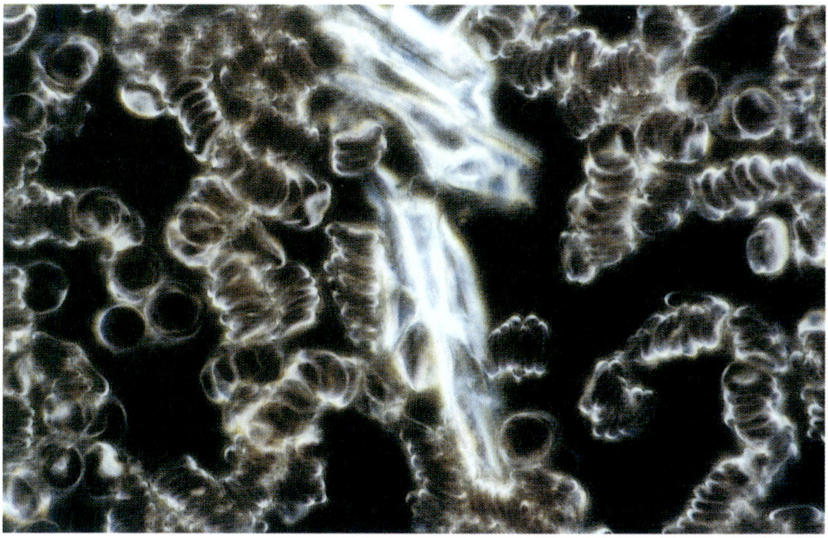

Aufnahme von: 7/1990 – Photo taken: 7/1990

Bewertung: Gelb-weißliche Pseudokristalle – Hinweis auf Belastung im Oberbauch; extreme Agglutionation der Erythrozyten – Stauungen, Durchblutungsstörungen.

Evaluation: Yellow-whitish pseudocrystals – indication to stress in upper abdomen; extreme agglutination of erythrocytes – congestions, disturbances of blood supply.

Patientin:	J., geb. 1945
Diagnose:	Leber-Galle-Stau

Patient (female):	J., bom 1945
Diagnosis:	Blockage of liver and gall bladder

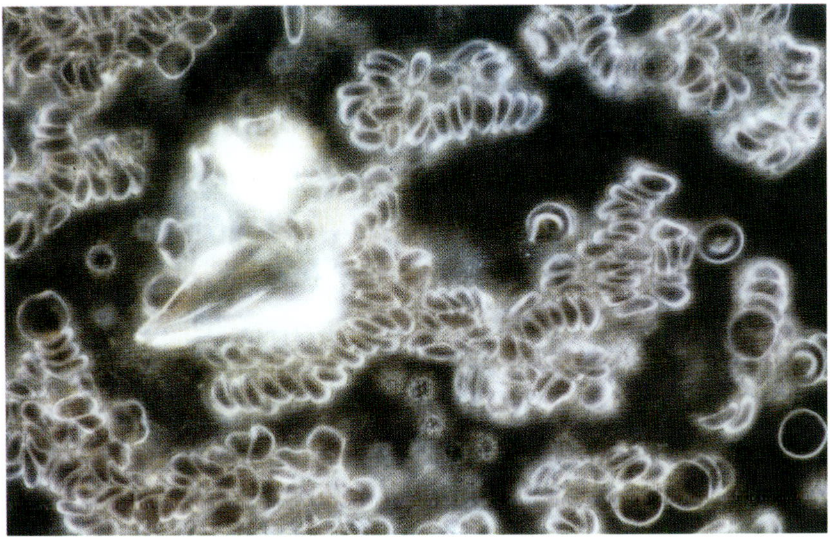

Aufnahme von: 1/1990 – Photo taken: 1/1990

Bewertung: Braune Pseudokristalle – Hinweis auf Oberbauch (Leber); starke Agglutination der Erythrozyten – Stauungen.

Evaluation: Brown pseudocrystals – indication to upper abdomen (liver); strong agglutination of erythrocytes – congestions.

Patientin:	M., geb. 1925
Diagnose:	Verdacht auf Cholezystitis, Pankreatitis

Patient (female):	M., born 1925
Diagnosis:	Suspected cholecystitis, pancreatitis

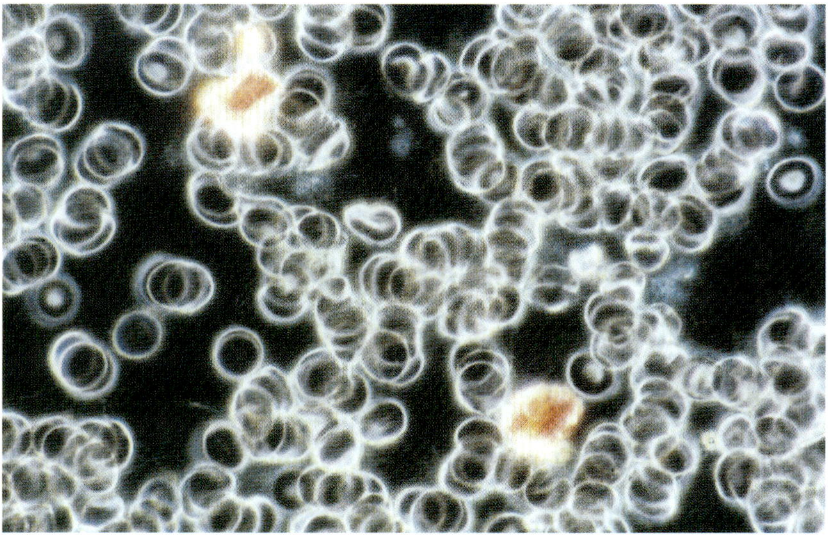

Aufnahme von: 1/1990 – Photo taken: 1/1990

Bewertung: Gelb-orange Pseudokristalle – Hinweis auf Oberbauch (Pankreas).

Evaluation: Yellow-orange pseudocrystals – indication to upper abdomen (pancreas).

Patient:	L., geb. 1922
Diagnose:	Pankreas-Galle-Magen-Syndrom, Gallengries, nervöser Magen

Patient:	L., born 1922
Diagnosis:	Syndrome of pancreas, gall and stomack, small gall-stones, nervous stomach

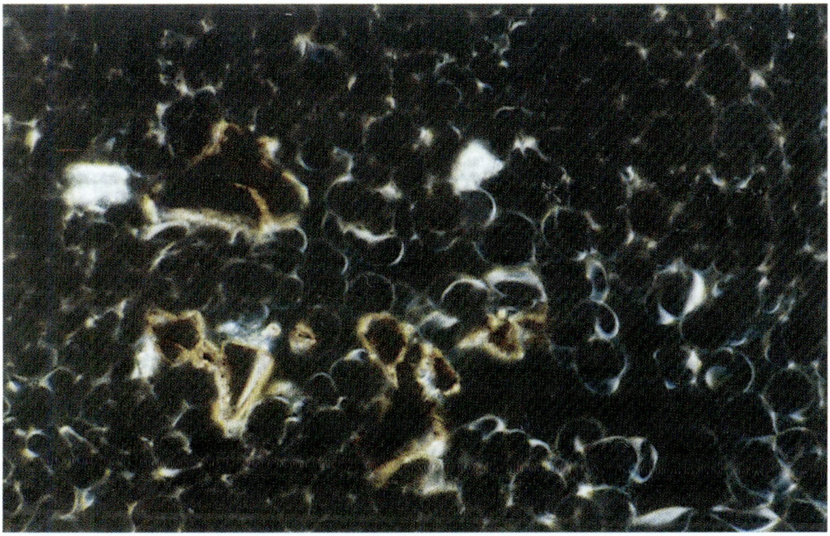

Aufnahme von: 6/1989 – Photo taken: 6/1989

Bewertung: Braun-gelbe Pseudokristalle – Hinweis auf Oberbauch (Leber); extreme Agglutination der Erythrozyten – Stauungen.

Evaluation: Brown-yellow pseudocrystals – indication to upper abdomen (liver); extreme agglutination of erythrocytes – congestions.

Patientin: F., geb. 1923
Diagnose: Colon-Ca, Coecum-Ca

Patient (female): L., born 1923
Diagnosis: Carcinoma of the colon, carcinoma of the cecum

Aufnahme 1 – Photo 1

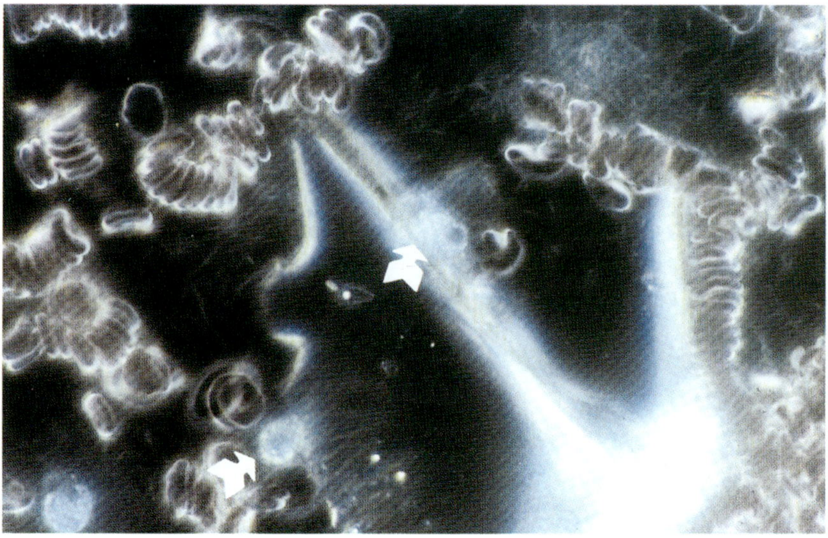

Aufnahme von: 7/1990 – Photo taken: 7/1990

Bewertung: Riesiges sklerotisches Gebilde – dunkle Farbe und Form Hinweis auf Leber; Form wird durch mehrere Leukozyten ➽ attackiert; extreme Agglutination der Erythrozyten, obere Bildhälfte Filitnest – Stauungen.

Evaluation: Massive sclerotic formation – dark colour and form, indication to liver; formation is being attacked by several leucocytes ➽; extreme agglutination of erythrocytes, filit nest in upper half of picture – congestions.

Patientin: F., geb. 1923
Diagnose: Colon-Ca, Coecum-Ca

Patient (female): L., born 1923
Diagnosis: Carcinoma of the colon, carcinoma of the cecum

Aufnahme 2 – Photo 2

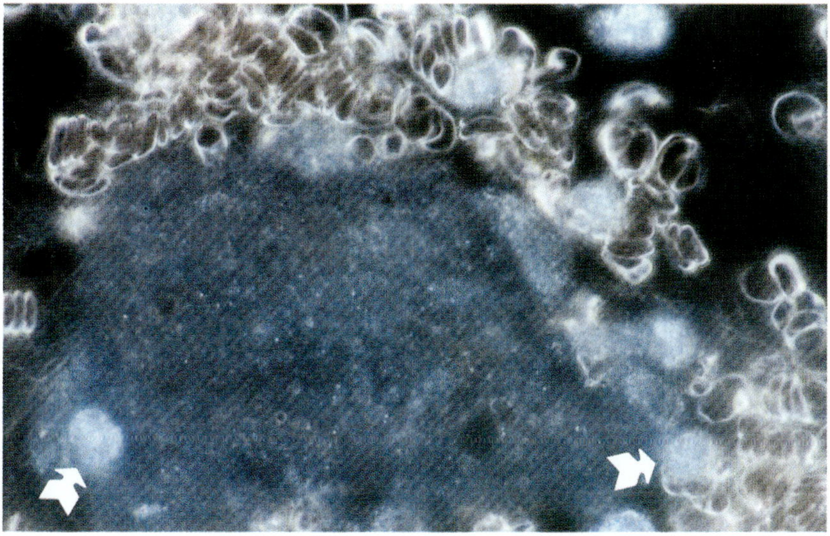

Aufnahme von: 7/1990 – Photo taken: 7/1990

B e w e r t u n g: Großer Symplast in Auflösung begriffen, von mehreren Granulozyten ➽ attackiert.

E v a l u a t i o n: Large symplast in state of degradation, attacked by several granulocytes ➽.

Patientin:	B., geb. 1964
Diagnose:	Asthma, Allergien, Sinusitis frontalis, Pyelonephritis

Patient (female):	B., born 1964
Diagnosis:	Asthma, allergies, sinusitis frontalis, pyelonephritis

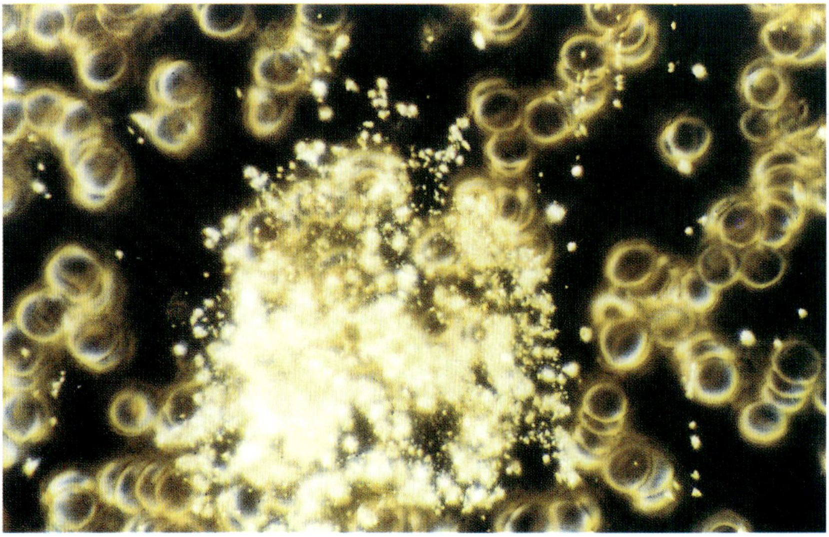

Aufnahme von: 12/1992 – Photo taken: 12/1992

Bewertung: Weiße Kristalle – Nierenbelastung

Evaluation: White crystals – kidney stress.

Patientin: S., geb. 1952
Diagnose: Neurodermitis, Verdacht auf Osteoporose, rechte Niere belastet

Patient (female): S., born 1952
Diagnosis: Neurodermitis, suspected osteoporosis, stress of right kidney

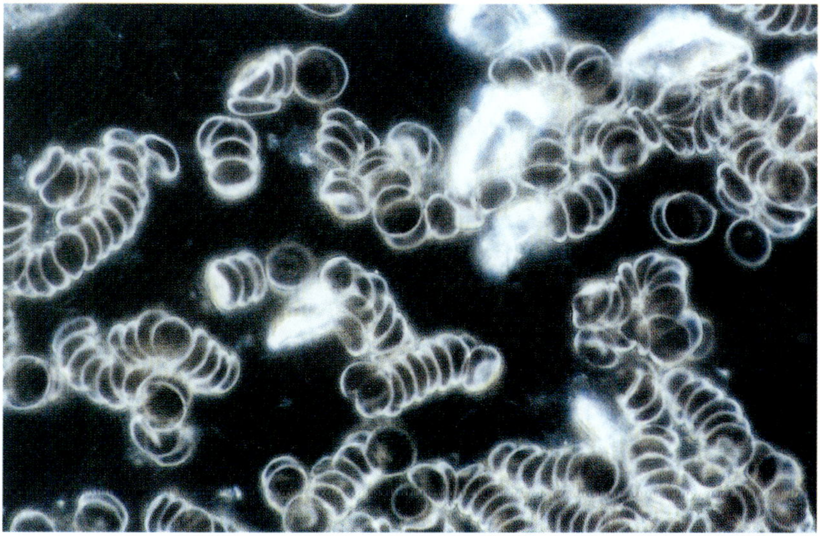

Aufnahme von: 4/1990 – Photo taken: 4/1990

Bewertung: Gelb-weiße Kristalle – Leberbelastung; Geldrollen, zum Teil gebogen – nach Prigge (1990) Darmbelastung, Endobiose.

Evaluation: Yellow-white crystals – liver stress; coin rolls, partly curved – according to Prigge (1990) intestinal stress, endobiosis.

Patientin: H., geb. 1937
Diagnose: Akuter Rheumaschub, urathische Diathese

Patient (female): H., born 1937
Diagnosis: Acute phase of rheumatism, uratic diathesis

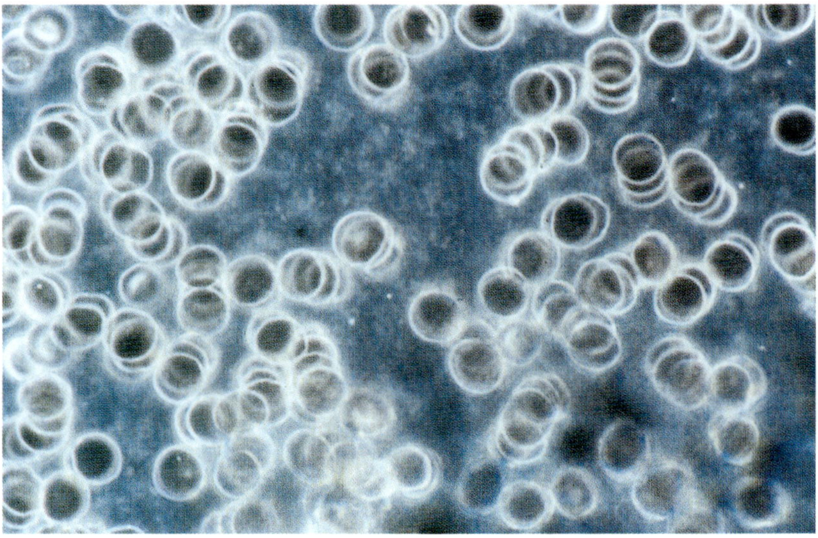

Aufnahme von: 6/1989 – Photo taken: 6/1989

Bewertung: Durch Überangebot von Eiweißkolloiden – Bildung von sklerotischen Formen im Blutplasma.

Evaluation: Through surplus of protein colloids – formation of sclerotic forms in the blood plasma.

Patientin: P., geb. 1908
Diagnose: Blasen-Ca, Durchblutungsstörungen in beiden Beinen, Gastritis, Colitis ulcerosa, Angina pectoris

Patient (female): P., born 1908
Diagnosis: Carcinoma of the bladder, disturbances of blood supply in both legs, gastritis, ulcerous colitis, angina pectoris

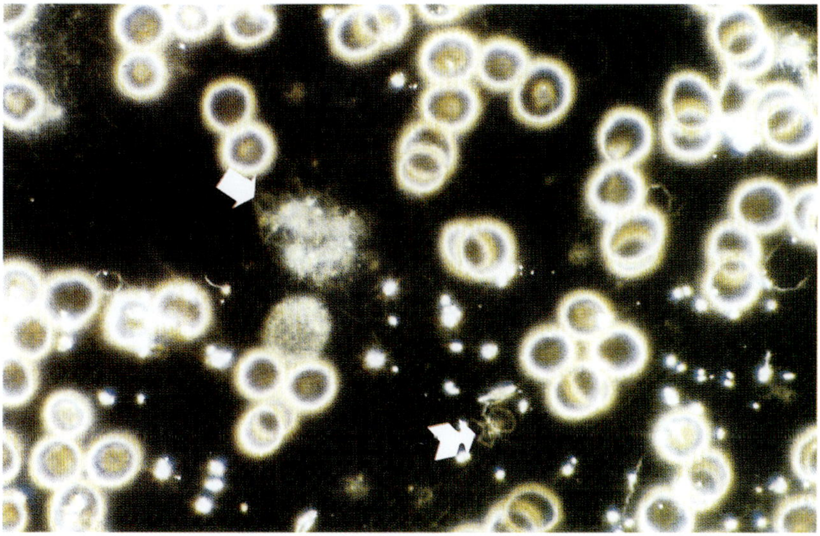

Aufnahme von: 1/1993 – Photo taken: 1/1993

Bewertung: Pteroharpe (➽) – Hinweis auf hohe Endobiose; in linker Bildhälfte ➡ Leukozyt, der in Chondrit-Dendroide zerfällt; unter dem Leukozyten ein, Lymphozyt, der von sporoiden Symprotiten befallen ist – zelluläre Abwehr stark geschwächt (1 h nach Blutentnahme).

Evaluation: Pteroharpe (➽) – indication to strong endobiosis; in the left half of the picture ➡ leucocyte which is degrading into chondrit-dendroids; below the leucocyte a lymphocyte which is infested with sporoid symprotits – cellular defence strongly weakened (one hour after taking a blood sample).

Patientin: H., geb. 1949
Diagnose: Colon-Ca (November 1991 OP)

Patient (female): H., born 1949
Diagnosis: Carcinoma of the colon (operation in November 1991)

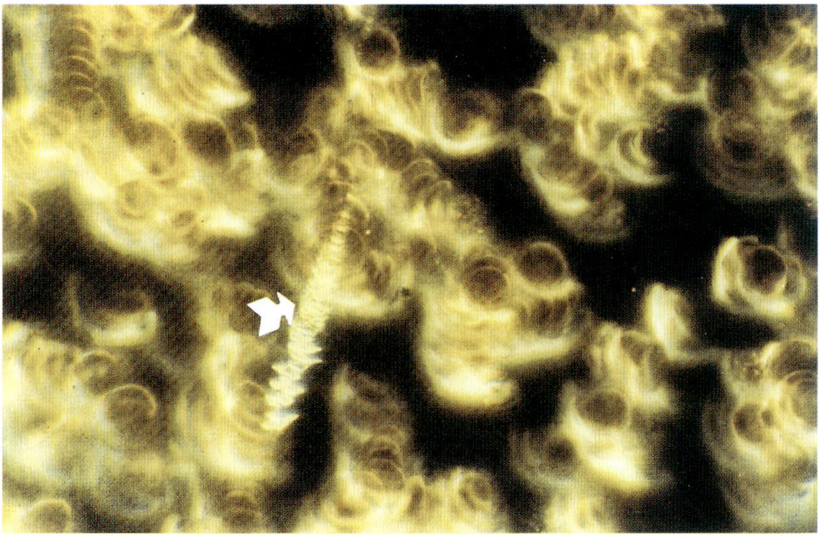

Aufnahme von: 7/1992 – Photo taken: 7/1992

Bewertung: ➽ In der Bildmitte Drepanide – Anzeichen für höhere Endobiose; starke Agglutination der Erythrozyten, Blutbild mit unscharfen Konturen – schweres Krankheitsbild.

Evaluation: ➽ In the centre of the picture drepanid – a sign of higher endobiosis; strong agglutination of the erythrocytes, blood picture with blurred contours – severe pathological picture.

Patient: W., geb. 1956, † 1991
Diagnose: Aids, Gliablastom

Patient: W., born 1956, † 1991
Diagnosis: Aids, gliablastom

Aufnahme 1 – Photo 1

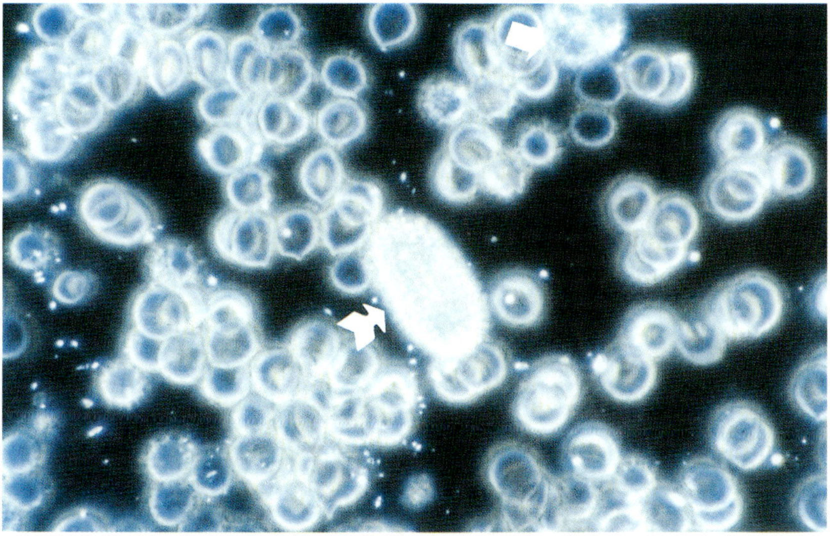

Aufnahme von: 9/1988 – Photo taken: 9/1988

Bewertung: ➽ Derosynascit mit kurzen stachelartigen Fortsätzen – hochpathogene Form; starke Endobiose der Erythrozyten (zitronenförmige E., Stechapfelformen, E. mit Chondriten);
➡ Leukozyt am oberen Bildrand befallen mit sporoiden Symprotiten, im Blutplasma sporoide Symprotite – schwere Endobiose.

Evaluation: ➽ Derosynascite with short thorn-like processes – highly pathogenic form; strong endobiosis of the erythrocytes (lemon-shaped erythrocytes, thorn-apple forms, erythrocytes with chondrits)
➡ leucocyte in the higher edge of the picture infested with sporoid symprotits, sporoid symprotits in the blood plasma – severe endobiosis.

Patien:	W., geb. 1956, † 1991
Diagnose:	Aids, Gliablastom
Patient:	W., born 1956, † 1991
Diagnosis:	Aids, gliablastom

Aufnahme 2 – Photo 2

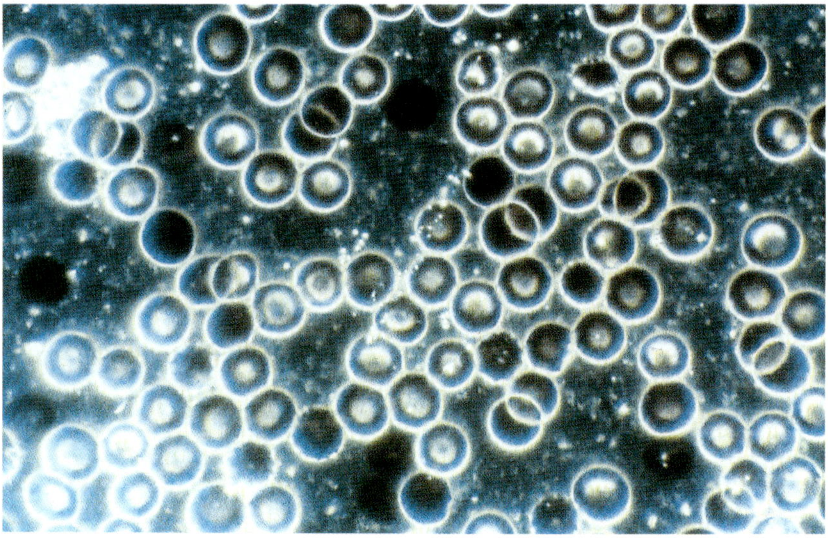

Aufnahme von: 9/1988 – Photo taken: 9/1988

Bewertung: Erythrozyten endobiontisch befallen, im Blutplasma grauer Niederschlag von zahlreichen sklerotischen Eiweißkolloiden – schweres Krankheitsbild.

Evaluation: Erythrocytes endobiontically infested, grey precipitates of numerous sclerotic protein colloids in the blood plasma – severe pathological picture.

Patientin: H., geb. 1937
Diagnose: Bauchraum-Ca mit Knochenmetastasen (Chemotherapie)

Patient (female): H., born 1937
Diagnosis: Carcinoma of the abdominal region with bone metastases (chemotherapy)

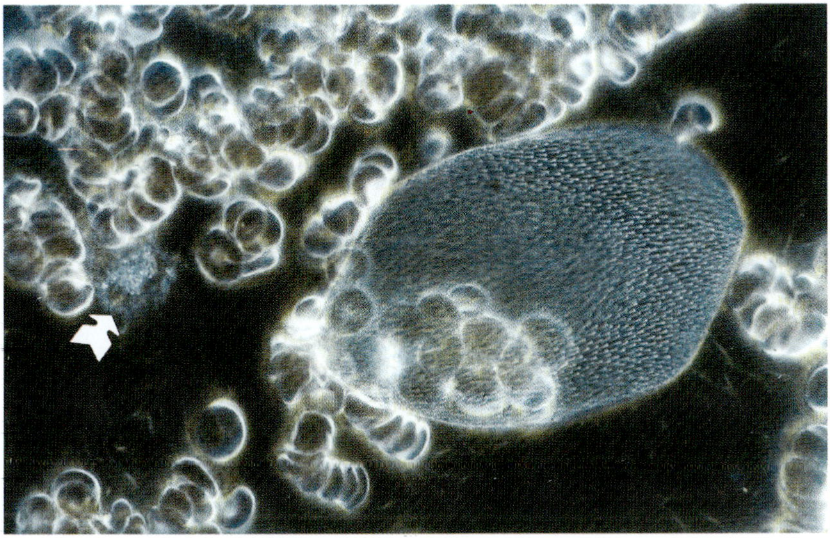

Aufnahme von: 10/1990 – Photo taken: 10/1990

Bewertung: Sklerotisches Gebilde mit zottenähnlichen Fortsätzen; Agglutination der Erythrozyten – Stauungen; linke Bildmitte zerfallender Leukozyt (➽) – zelluläre Abwehr geschwächt; schwache Filitbildung im Plasma.

Evaluation: Sclerotic formation with villi-like processes; agglutination of the erythrocytes – congestions; left centre of the picture leucocyte (➽) in state of degradation – weakened cellular defence; slight filit formation in the plasma.

Patientin:	H., geb. 1923, † 1990
Diagnose:	Nierenkrebs, urathische Diathese

Patient (female):	H., born 1923, † 1990
Diagnosis:	Cancer of the kidney, urathic diathesis

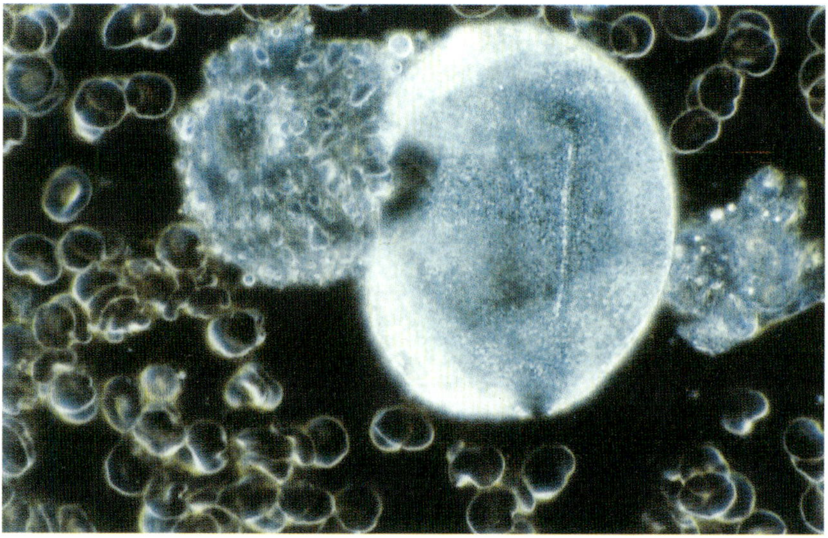

Aufnahme von: 8/1988 – Photo taken: 8/1988

Bewertung: Nierenähnliches sklerotisches Gebilde – schweres Krankheitsbild.

Evaluation: Sclerotic formation resembling a kidney – severe pathological picture.

Patient:	A., geb. 1925
Diagnose:	Urathische Diathese

Patient:	A., born 1925
Diagnosis:	Urathic diathesis

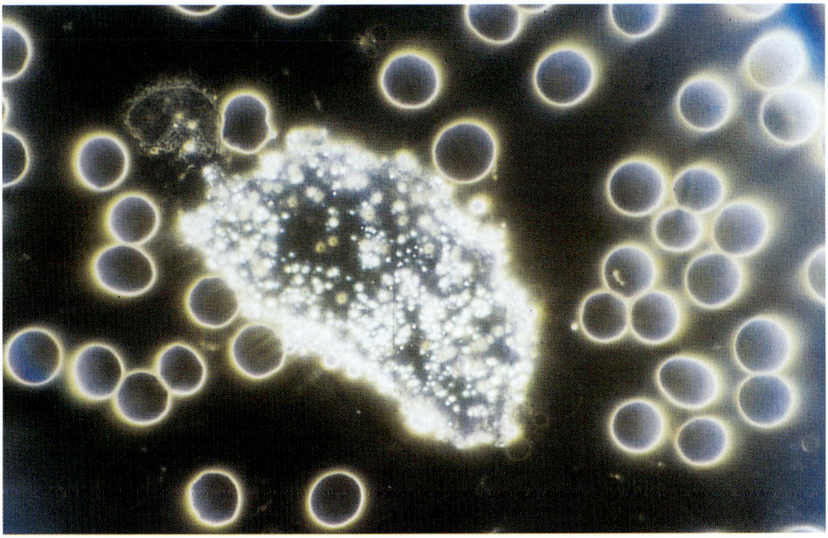

Aufnahme von: 3/1995 – Photo taken: 3/1995

Bewertung: Symplast mit sporoiden Symprotiten – Nierenbelastung oder urathische Diathese.

Evaluation: Symplast with sporoid symprotits – kidney stress or urathic diathesis.

Patientin: St., geb. 1952
Diagnose: Chronische Sinusitis generalis, Nieren- und Gallenkoliken, Angina pectoris, Herzmuskelschwäche, Apoplex, früher Gichtanfälle, Pyelonephritis

Patient (female): St., born 1952
Diagnosis: Chronic sinusitis generalis, kidney and gall-stone colics, angina pectoris, myocardiac weakness, apoplexia, earlier attacks of gout, pyelonephritis

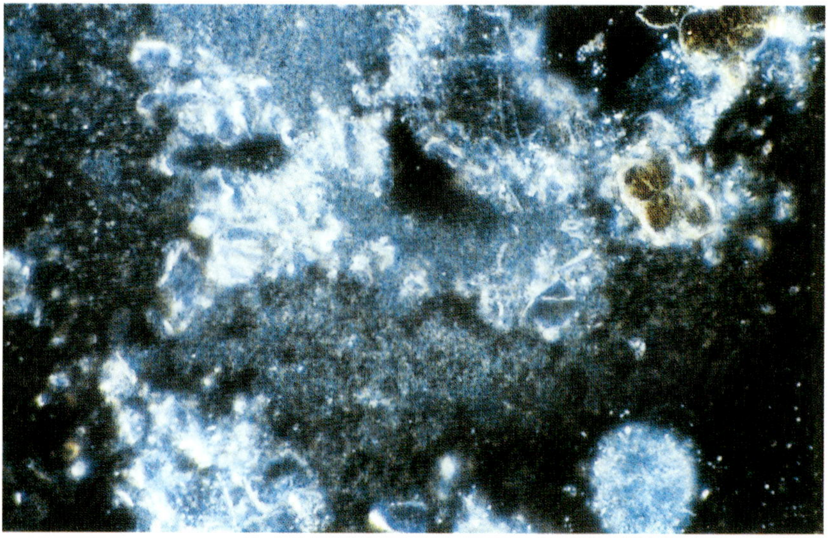

Aufnahme von: 1/1990 – Photo taken: 1/1990

Bewertung: Riesige Ansammlung von sklerotischen Parasitengebilden (Pseudokristalle, die auf Leber- und Nierenbelastung hinweisen) – schweres Krankheitsbild (12 h nach Blutentnahme).

Evaluation: Huge accumulation of sclerotic parasitic formations (pseudocrystals that indicate to liver and kidney stress) – severe pathological picture (12 hours after taking a blood sample).

Patientin: S., geb. 1925
Diagnose: Colitis ulcerosa, Durchblutungsstörungen

Patient (female): S., born 1925
Diagnosis: Ulcerous colitis, disturbances of blood supply

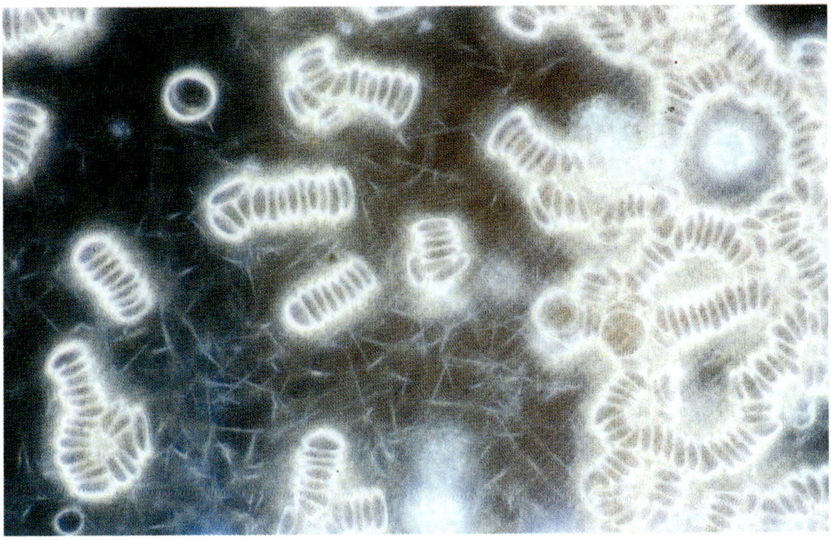

Aufnahme von: 2/1990 – Photo taken: 2/1990

Bewertung: Starke Agglutination der Erythrozyten – Bewegungseinschränkung der E. mit der Folge von Stauungen und Durchblutungsstörungen, Sauerstoffunterversorgung der Zellen; gebogene Geldrollen – nach Prigge (1990) Darmbelastung; Filite im Plasma – erhöhte Fibrinbildung, Stauungen, Übersäuerung des Bindegewebes.

Evaluation: Strong agglutination of erythrocytes – restricted movements of erythrocytes with the consequences of congestions and disturbances of blood supply, inadequate supply of oxygen to the cells, curved coin rolls – according to Prigge (1990) intestinal stress; filits in the plasma – increased fibrin formation, congestions, overascidification of the connective tissue.

Patient: A., geb. 1942
Diagnose: Chronische Polyarthritis, chronische Sinusitis

Patient: A., born 1942
Diagnosis: Chronic polyarthritis, chronic sinusitis

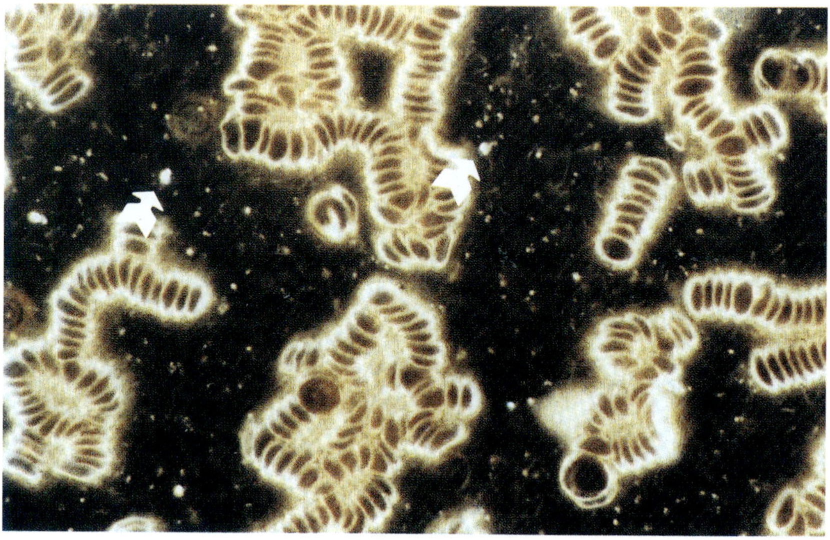

Aufnahme von: 9/1992 – Photo taken: 9/1992

Bewertung: Geldrollenbildung – Endobiose; schwache Filitbildung im Plasma – Stauungen; ➽ vereinzelt Makrosymprotite im Plasma – „Mucor-Belastung".

Evaluation: Coin roll formation – endobiosis; weak filit formation in the plasma – congestions; ➽ scattered macrosymprotits in the plasma – „Mucor-burden".

Patient: H., geb. 1931
Diagnose: Herzinfarkt, Apoplex, harnsaure Diathese, Gicht

Patient: H., born 1931
Diagnosis: Cardiac infarction, apoplexia, uric acid diathesis, gout

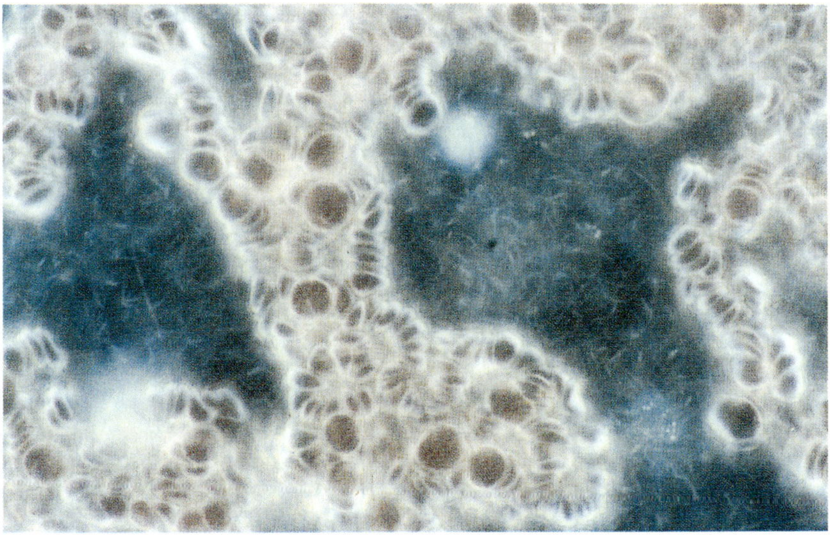

Aufnahme von: 2/1990 – Photo taken: 2/1990

Bewertung: Extreme Aggregation der Erythrozyten – Stauungen, Durchblutungsstörungen; starke Filitbildung – Stauungen, Übersäuerung.

Evaluation: Extreme aggregation of erythrocytes – congestions, disturbances of blood supply; strong filit formation – congestions, acidosis.

Patient: K., geb. 1927
Diagnose: Mesotheliom

Patient: K., born 1927
Diagnosis: Mesotheliom

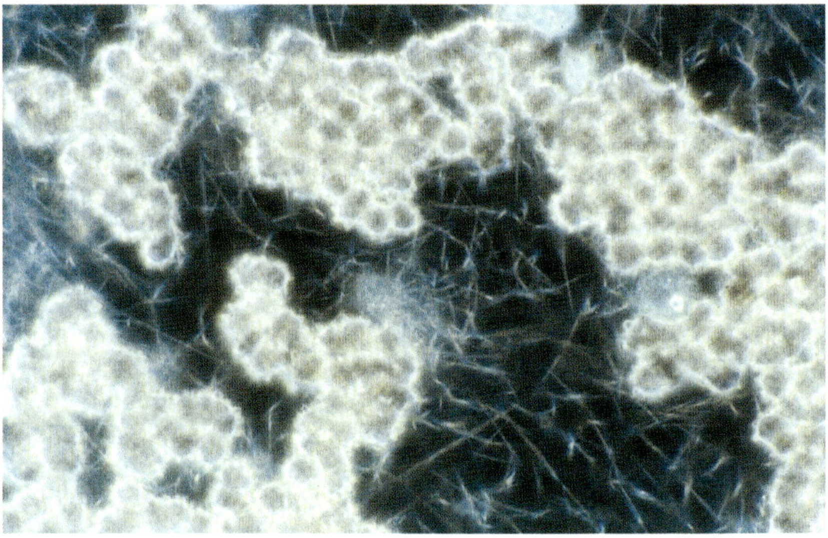

Aufnahme von: 8/1989 – Photo taken: 8/1989

Bewertung: Erythrozyten endobiontisch stark belastet, extreme Agglutination – Einschränkung der Funktionsfähigkeit der E. mit der Folge von Stauungen, Durchblutungsstörungen und Sauerstoffdefizit, schwere Endobiose; Filitbildung im Plasma – Stauungen.

Evaluation: Erythrocytes with strong endobiontic burden, extreme agglutination – restricted function of mobility of the erythrocytes with the consequence of congestions, disturbances of blood supply and deficiency of oxygen; severe endobiosis; filit formation in the plasma – congestions.

Patientin: M., geb. 1937
Diagnose: Chronische Sinusitis frontalis, Bronchitis, Klimakterium, Hämorrhoiden

Patient (female): M., born 1937
Diagnosis: Chronic sinusitis frontalis, bronchitis, climacteric, hemorrhoids

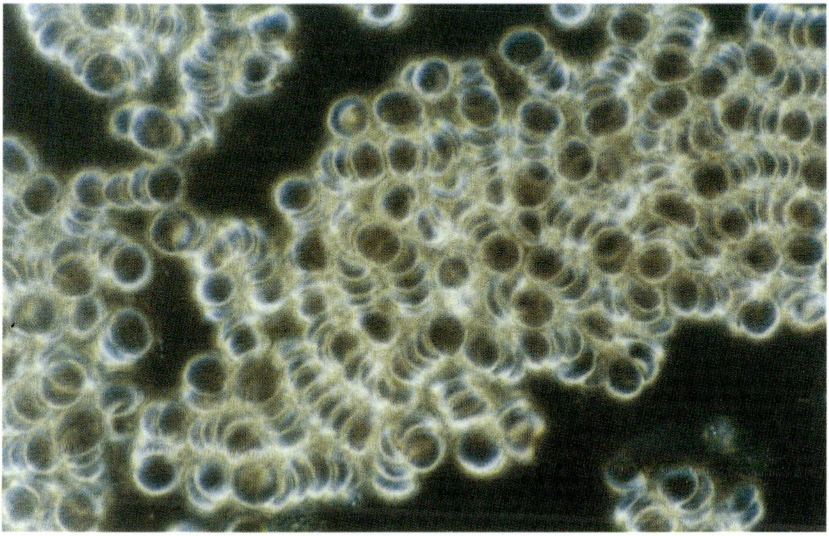

Aufnahme von: 2/1989 – Photo taken: 2/1989

Bewertung: Agglutination der Erythrozyten – Durchblutungsstörungen, Entgleisung der Mucor-Zyklode; kaum Spermiten und Symprotite im Plasma – symbiontische Abwehr geschwächt.

Evaluation: Agglutination of the erythrocytes disturbances of bloods supply, derailment of the Mucor-cyclode; hardly any spermits and symprotits in the plasma – symbiontic defence weakened.

Patient: B., geb. 1909
Diagnose: Arteriosklerose, Katarakt links, Hörsturz links

Patient: B., born 1909
Diagnosis: Arteriosclerosis, cataract of the left eye, auditory fall left

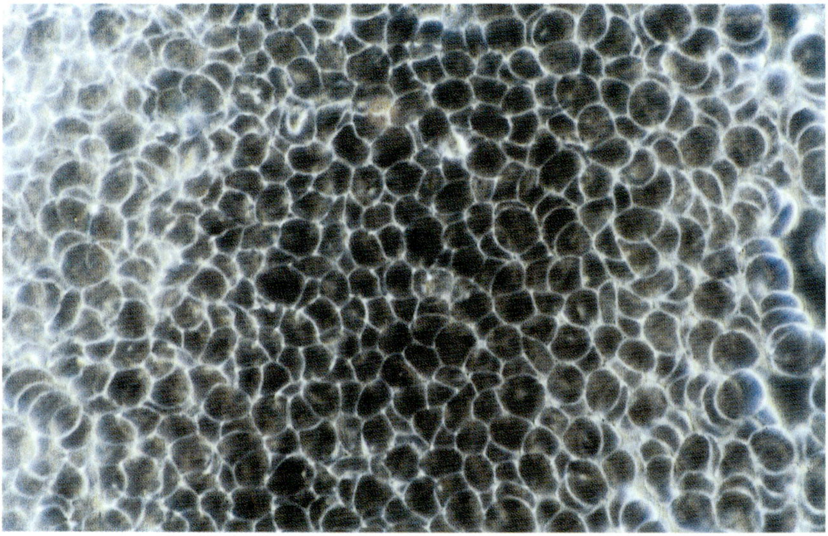

Aufnahme von: 2/1989 – Photo taken: 2/1989

Bewertung: Extreme Agglutination der Erythrozyten in Form eines Erythrozyten-Thrombus – schwere Endobiose.

Evaluation: Extreme agglutination of the erythrocytes under the form of an erythrocyte thrombus – severe endobiosis.

Patient: H., geb. 1938
Diagnose: Hochgradige Verengung der beiden Halsschlagadern, Apoplex 1988, Durchblutungsstörungen im Lendenwirbelbereich

Patient : H., born 1938
Diagnosis: Extreme stricture of both carotid arteries, apoplexia 1988, disturbances of blood supply in the lumbar vertebra region

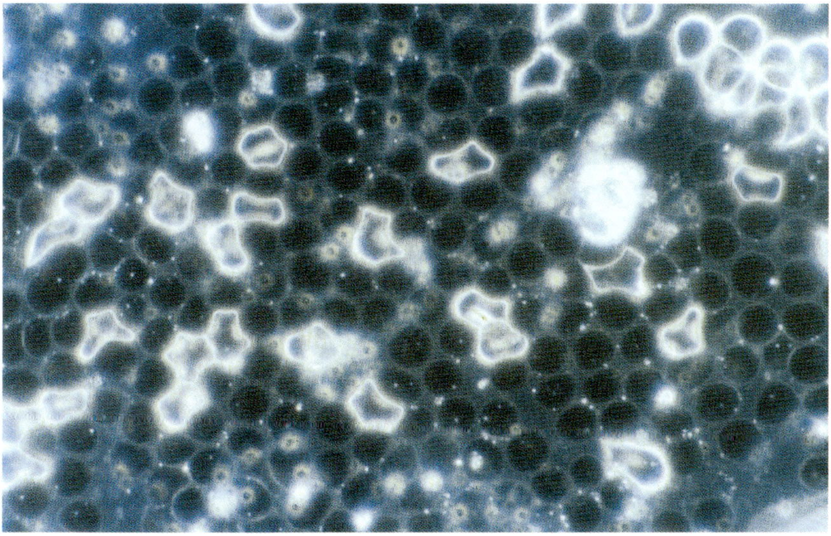

Aufnahme von: 2/1990 – Photo taken: 2/1990

Bewertung: Erythrozyten-Thrombus mit schwarzen Erythrozyten (Blutschatten) – schwere Endobiose.

Evaluation: Erythrocyte thrombus with black erythrocytes (blood shadows) – severe endobiosis.

Patient: Sch., geb. 1930
Diagnose: Teilweiser Verschluß der beiden Oberschenkelarterien

Patient: Sch., born 1930
Diagnosis: Partial obturation of both femoral arteries

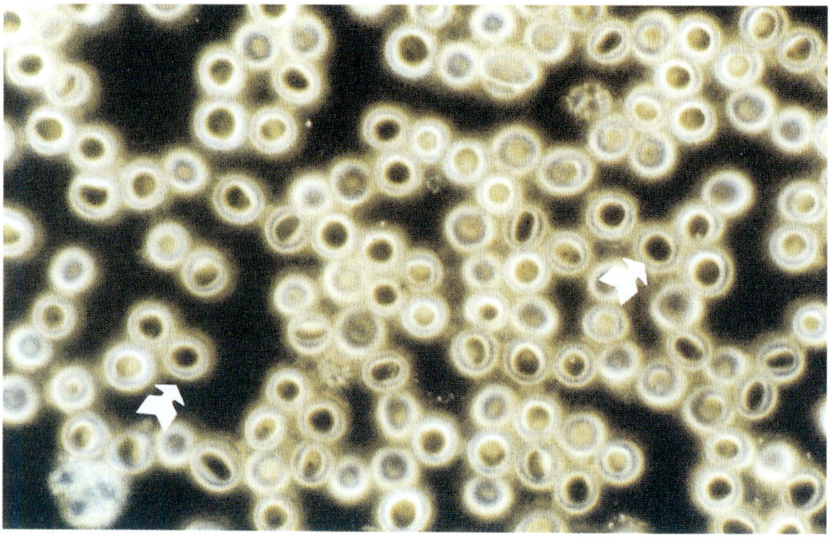

Aufnahme von: 12/1992 – Photo taken: 12/1992

Bewertung: ➽ „Schießscheibenerythrozyten" – Endobiose; wenig Symbionten im Plasma – Abwehrschwache.

Evaluation: ➽ „Target erythrocytes" – endobiosis; few symbionts in the plasma – defence weakness.

Patient: P., geb. 1955
Diagnose: Chronische Sinusitis, Otitis, Sodbrennen, Psoriasis

Patient: P., born 1955
Diagnosis: Chronic sinusitis, otitis, heartburn, psoriasis

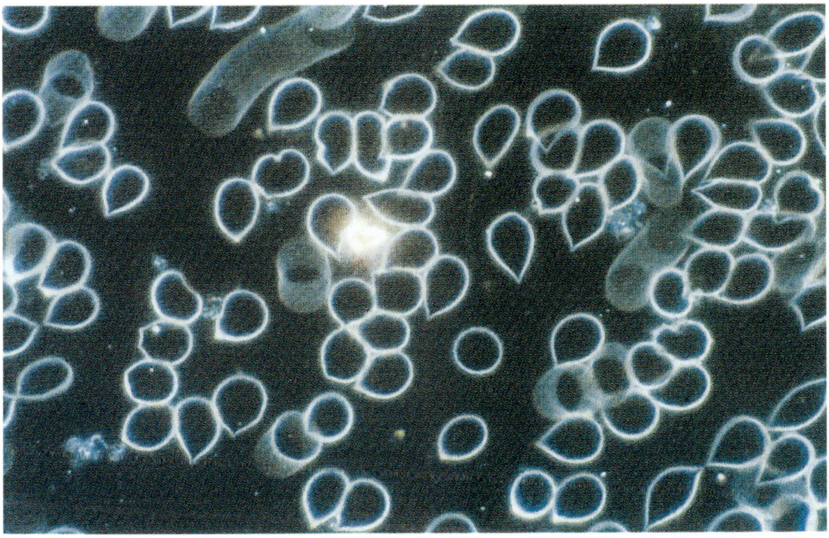

Aufnahme von: 5/1989 – Photo taken: 5/1989

Bewertung: Zitronenförmige Erythrozyten, in der Bildmitte Kristall – Leberbelastung.

Evaluation: Lemon-shaped erythrocytes, in the centre of the picture crystal – liver stress.

Patient: P., geb. 1955
Diagnose: Chronische Sinusitis, Otitis, Sodbrennen, Psoriasis

Patient: P., born 1955
Diagnosis: Chronic sinusitis, otitis, heartburn, psoriasis

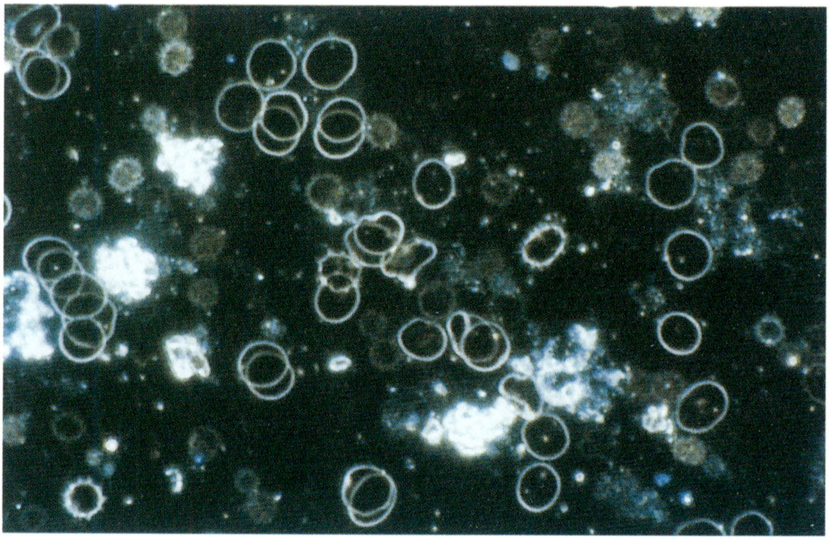

Aufnahme von: 5/1989 – Photo taken: 5/1989

Bewertung: „Schwarzes Loch" = dunkle Stelle mit zahlreichen endobiontisch schwer belasteten Erythrozyten – Hinweis auf Entzündungsherd im Körper; weiße Kristalle – Hinweis auf Nierenbelastung.

Evaluation: „Black hole" = dark spot with numerous, endobiontically severely burdened erythrocytes – indication to an inflammatory focus in the body; white crystals – indication to kidney stress.

Patientin: C., geb. 1932
Diagnose: Leber-Galle-Stau, Dickdarmstau, Sodbrennen

Patient (female): C., born 1932
Diagnosis: Liver-gall congestion, colon congestion, heartburn

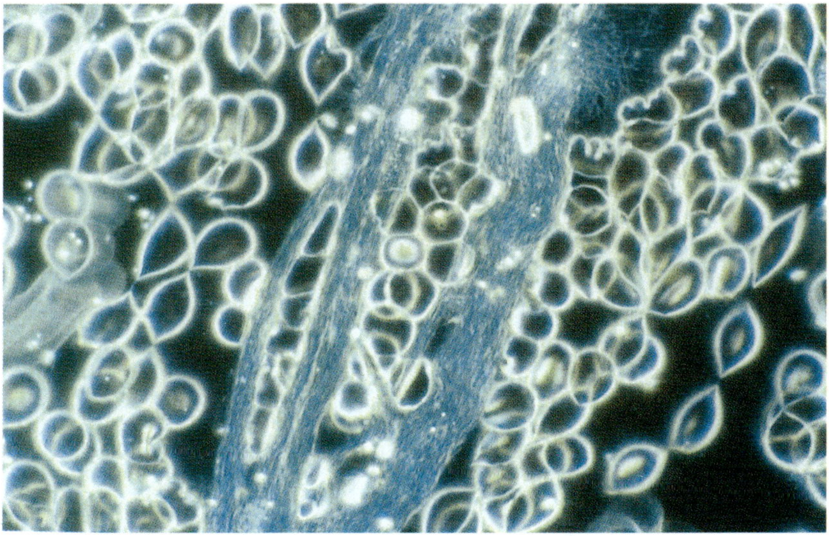

Aufnahme von: 8/1988 – Photo taken: 8/1988

Bewertung: Zitronenförmige Erythrozyten, in Ketten angeordnet, in Bildmitte entstehender Symplast – schwere Leberbelastung, Endobiose.

Evaluation: Lemon-shaped erythrocytes in chain formation, in the centre of the picture developing symplast – strong liver stress, endobiosis.

Patientin: A., geb. 1955
Diagnose: Eisenmangelanämie

Patient (female): A., born 1955
Diagnosis: Anemia

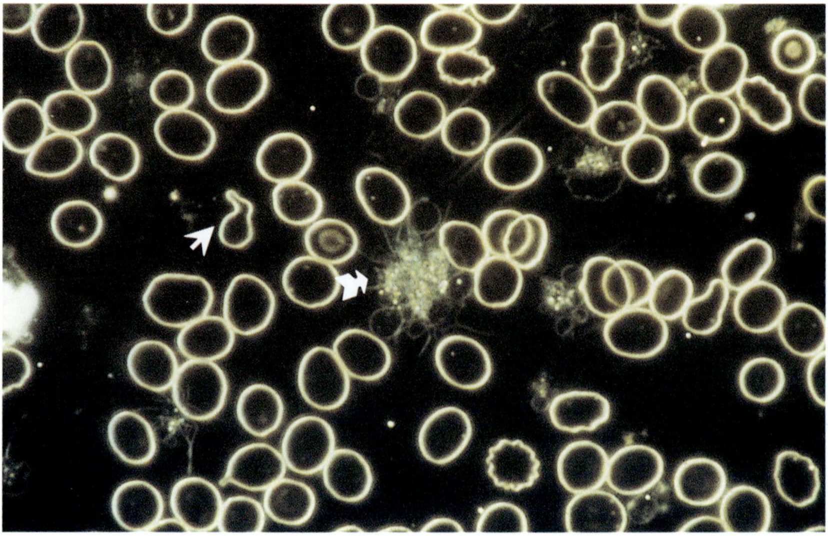

Aufnahme von: 2/1999 – Photo taken: 2/1999

Bewertung: ➚ Erythrozyt mit herauswachsendem Bakterienstäbchen (Leptotrichia buccalis) – Endobiose;
➚ in der Mitte zerfallener Leukozyt mit Kolloidtheciten – geschwächte zelluläre Abwehr.

Evaluation: ➚ Erythrocyte with exuding bacterial rod (Leptotrichia buccalis) – endobiosis;
➚ in the centre leucocyte in state of degradation with kolloid-thecites – weakened cellular defence.

Patientin: M., geb. 1942
Diagnose: Rheumatische Gelenkbeschwerden mit Beteiligung der Nieren

Patient (female): M., born 1942
Diagnosis: Rheumatic joint troubles with implication of the kidneys

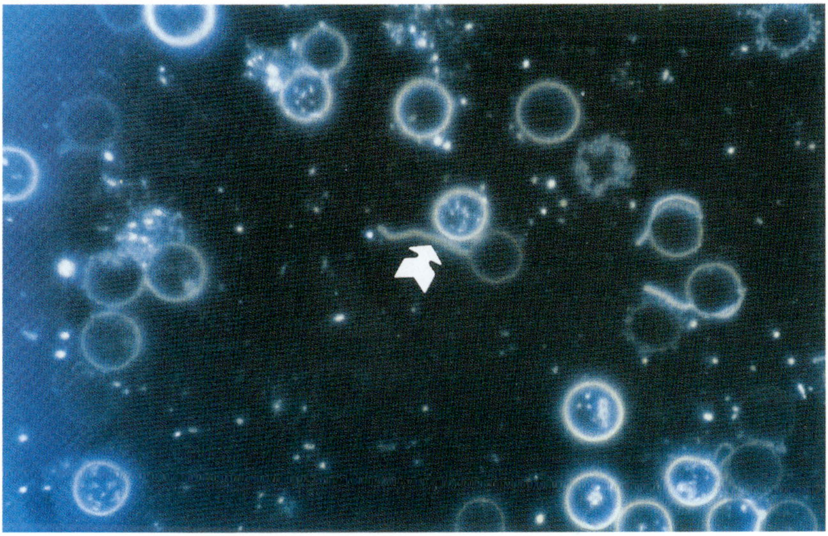

Aufnahme von: 8/1990 – Photo taken: 8/1990

Bewertung: Endobiontischer Befall der Erythrozyten, teilweise mit Bildung von Bakterienstäbchen ➽ – beginnende Freisetzung der Erreger, Lösung der Blockade (Mochlolyse) durch die Therapie (nach 2 h).

Evaluation: Endobiontic infestation of the erythrocytes, partly with the formation of bacterial rods ➽ – starting release of the pathogens, unblocking (mochlolysis) by means of the therapy (after 2 hours).

Patient:	Sch., geb. 1945
Diagnose:	Angina pectoris

Patient:	Sch., born 1945
Diagnosis:	Angina pectoris

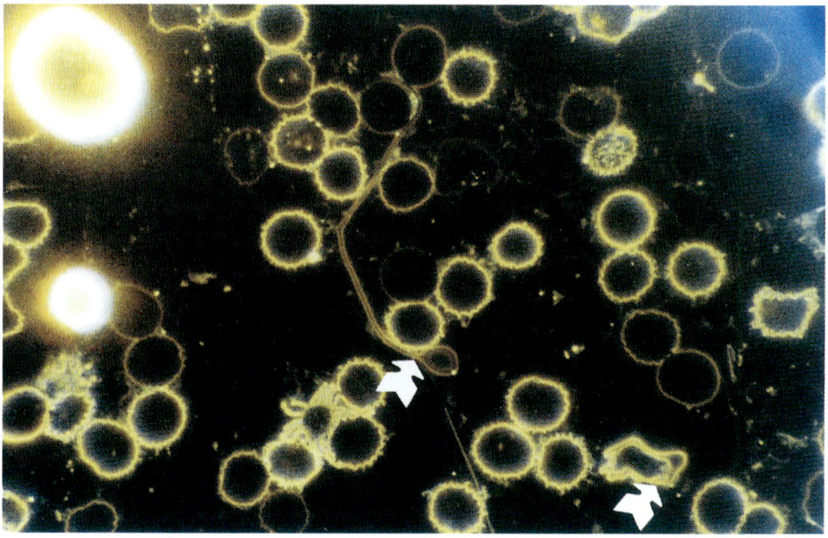

Aufnahme von: 3/1993 – Photo taken: 3/1993

Bewertung: ➽ Erythrozyten mit herauswachsenden Bakterienstäbchen des Endobionten – schwere Endobiose (1 h nach Blutabnahme).

Evaluation: ➽ Erythrocytes with exuding bacterial rods of the endobiont (one hour after taking a blood sample) – strong endobiosis.

Patientin: A., geb. 1955
Diagnose: Eisenmangelanämie

Patient (female): A., born 1995
Diagnosis: Anemia

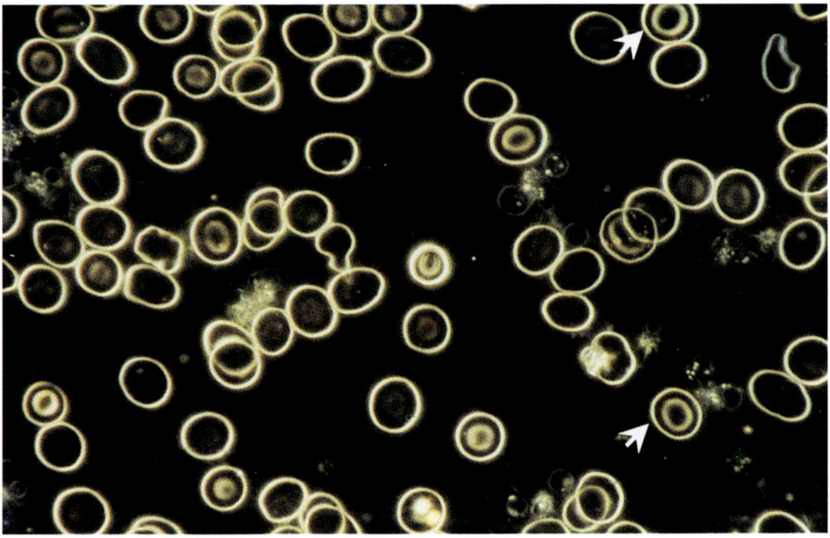

Aufnahme von: 4/1999 – Photo taken: 4/1999

Bewertung: Anisozytose (Größenverschiedenheit der Erythrozyten) – Eisenmangelanämie;
➚ Targetzellen – verschiedene Anämieformen.

Evaluation: Anisocytosis – anemia:
➚ Target erythrocytes – different forms of anemia.

Patientin: G., geb. 1975
Diagnose: Angina lacunaris, Fieber, Allergien, Neurodermitis, Herpes labialis

Patient (female): G., born 1975
Diagnosis: Lacunar angina, fever, allergies, neurodermitis, labial herpes

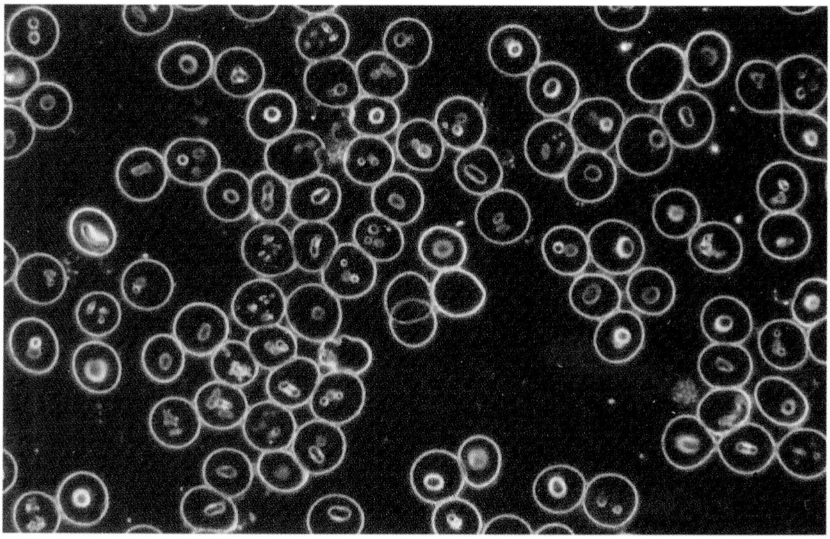

Aufnahme von: 8/1989 – Photo taken: 8/1989

Bewertung: Starker endobiontischer Befall der Erythrozyten; starke Lumineszenz der Erythrozytenmembranen – nach Prigge (1990) Energieschwäche der Erythrozyten.

Evaluation: Heavy endobiontic infestation of the erythrocytes; strong luminescence of the membranes of the erythrocytes – according to Prigge (1990) weakness of energy of the erythrocytes.

Patient: K., geb. 1917, † 1990
Diagnose: Colon-Ca mit Lebermetastasen

Patient: K., born 1917, † 1990
Diagnosis: Carcinoma of the colon with liver metastasises

Aufnahme 1 – Photo 1

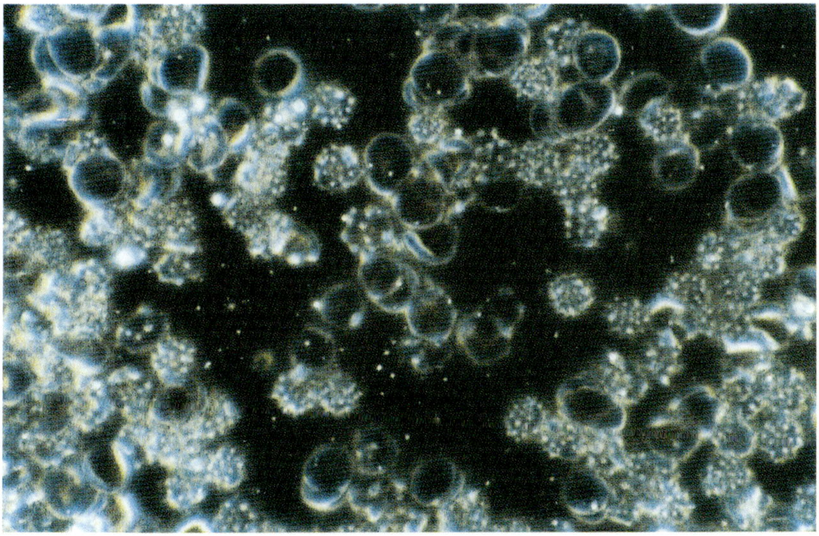

Aufnahme vom 5/1989 Photo taken: 5/1989

Bewertung: Erythrozyten mit sporoiden Symprotiten – hohe endobiontische Belastung.

Evaluation: Erythrocytes with sporoid symprotits – high endobiontic burden.

Patient:	K., geb. 1917, † 1990
Diagnose:	Colon-Ca mit Lebermetastasen

Patient:	K., born 1917, † 1990
Diagnosis:	Carcinoma of the colon with liver metastasises

Aufnahme 2 – Photo 2

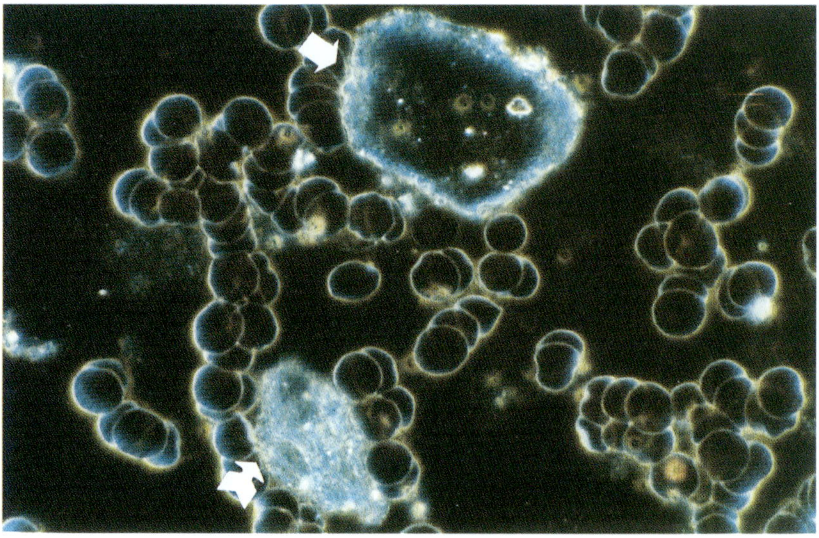

Aufnahme von: 5/1989 – Photo taken: 5/1989

Bewertung: ➽ „Aspergillus-" und ➡ Sklerosymplast; Agglutination der Erythrozyten – Endobiose; Plasma fast ohne Symprotite und Spermite – symbiontische Abwehr kommt zum Erliegen.

Evaluation: ➽ „Aspergillus symplast" and ➡ sclerosymplast; agglutination of erythrocytes – endobiosis; plasma almost without symprotits and spermits – symbiontic defence comes to a standstill.

Patient: B., geb. 1925
Diagnose: Osteomyosklerose

Patient: B., born 1925
Diagnosis: Osteomyosclerosis

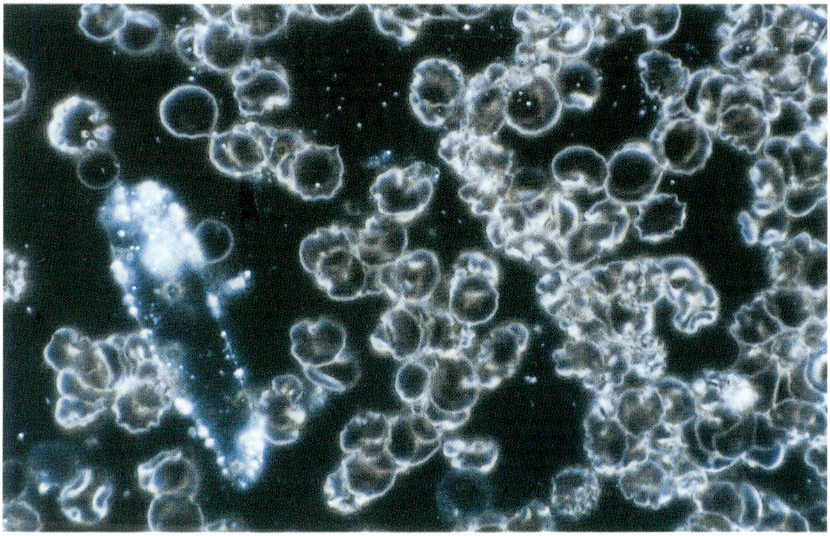

Aufnahme von: 1/1990 – Photo taken: 1/1990

Bewertung: Extreme Belastung der Erythrozyten – schwere Endobiose; unten links Sklerosymplast (20 Minuten nach Blutentnahme).

Evaluation: Erythrocytes extremely burdened – severe endobiosis; sclerosymplast below on the left (20 minutes after taking a blood sample).

Patient: P., geb. 1933
Diagnose: Galle-Leber-Stau, Hämorrhoiden, CWS-Syndrom, Gelenkbeschwerden

Patient: P., born 1933
Diagnosis: Gall-liver-blockage, hemorrhoids, CVS-syndrome, troubles of the joints

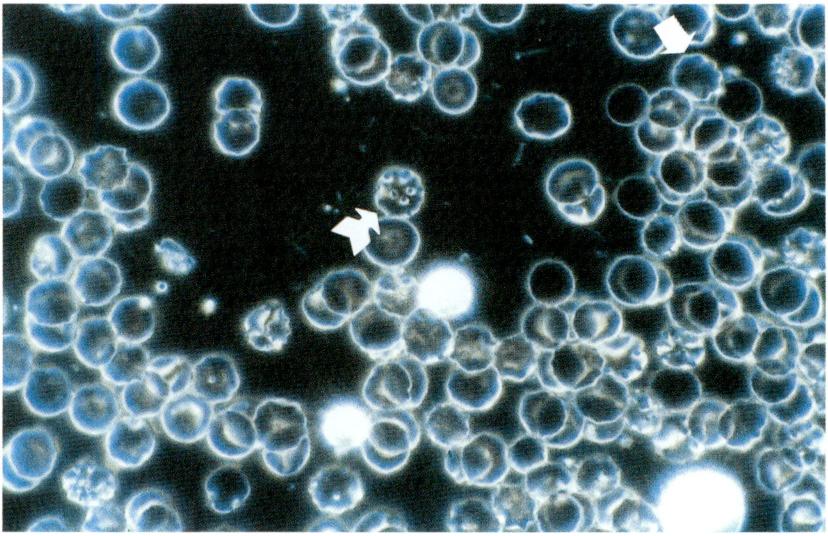

Aufnahme von: 9/1988 – Photo taken: 9/1988

Bewertung: Endobiontisch belastete Erythrozyten mit Vakuolen ➽
und Randzacken ➡ – „Mucor-Belastung".

Evaluation: Endobiontically burdened erythrocytes with vacuoles ➽
and marginal points ➡ – „Mucor burden".

Patientin: F., geb. 1945
Diagnose: Multiple Sklerose

Patient (female): F., born 1945
Diagnosis: Multiple sclerosis

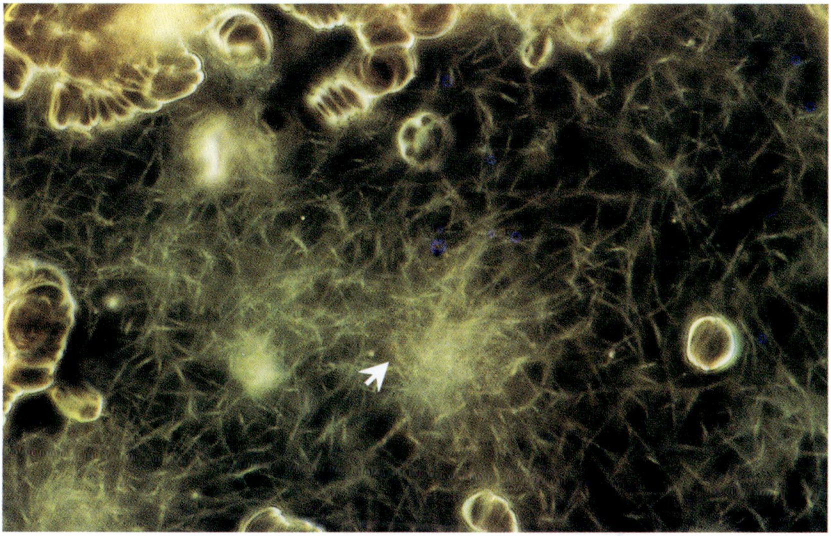

Aufnahme von: 3/1995 – Photo taken: 3/1995

Bewertung: ➚ In der Mitte Chondritdendroide aus zerfallenen Erythrozyten – schwere Endobiose; Geldrollen- und Filitbildung – Stauungen.

Evaluation: ➚ In the centre chondrit-dendroids from erythrocytes in state of degradation – severe endobiosis; coin roll formation and filites – congestions.

Patient: Sch., geb. 1945
Diagnose: Angina pectoris

Patient: Sch., born 1945
Diagnosis: Angina pectoris

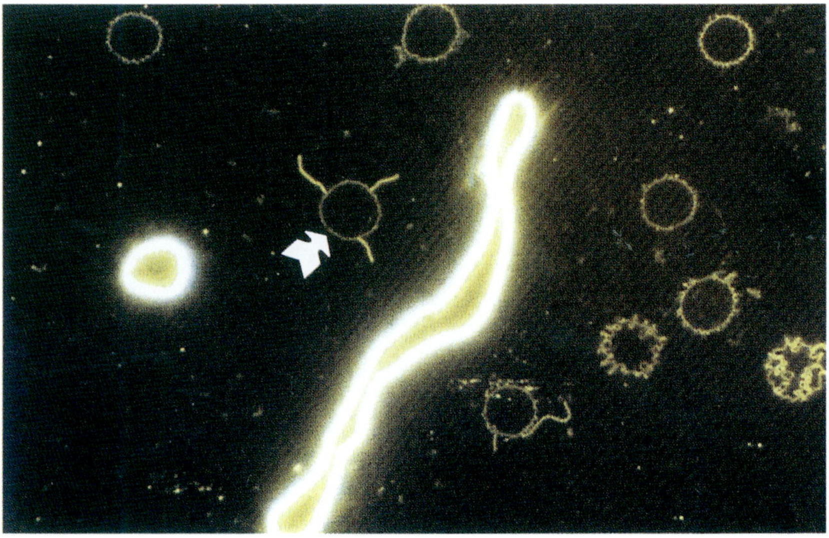

Aufnahme von: 6/1993 – Photo taken: 6/1993

Bewertung: ➽ Erythrozyten mit Chondriten – schwere Endobiose (2 h nach Blutentnahme).

Evaluation: ➽ Erythrocytes with chondrits – severe endobiosis (two hours after taking a blood sample).

Patientin: R., geb. 1945
Diagnose: Osteomyelosklerose

Patient (female): R., born 1945
Diagnosis: Osteomyelosclerosis

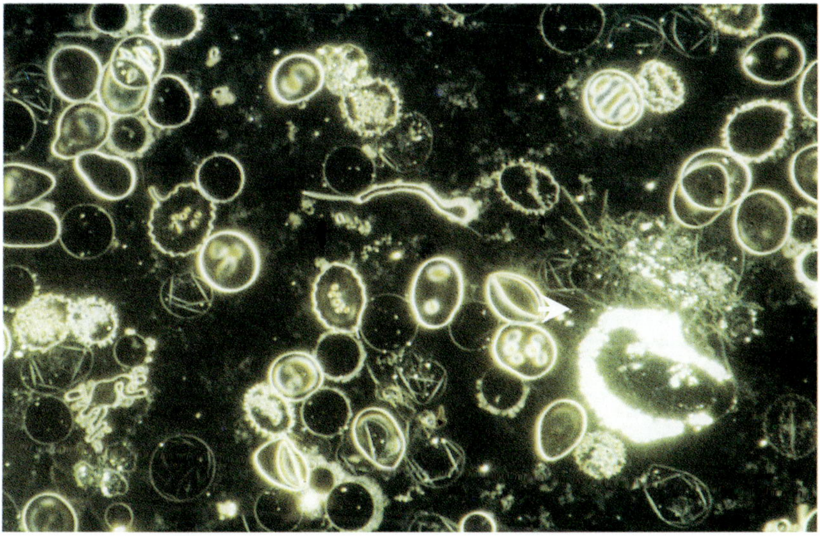

Aufnahme von: 4/1999 – Photo taken: 4/1999

B e w e r t u n g: Extremer endobiontischer Befall der Erythrozyten – schweres Krankheitsbild;
➔ 2 zerfallende Leukozyten, oberer mit Chrondritdendroiden – geschwächte zelluläre Abwehr (2 h nach Blutabnahme).

E v a l u a t i o n: Extreme endobiontic infestation of the erythrocytes – severe pathological picture;
➔ 2 leucocytes in state of degradation, leucocyte on the top with chrondrit-dendroides – weakened cellular defence (2 hour after taking a blood sample).

Leukozyten

Patient: W., geb. 1956, † 1991
Diagnose: AIDS, Glioblastom

Leucocytes

Patient: W., born 1956, † 1991
Diagnosis: AIDS, glioblastom

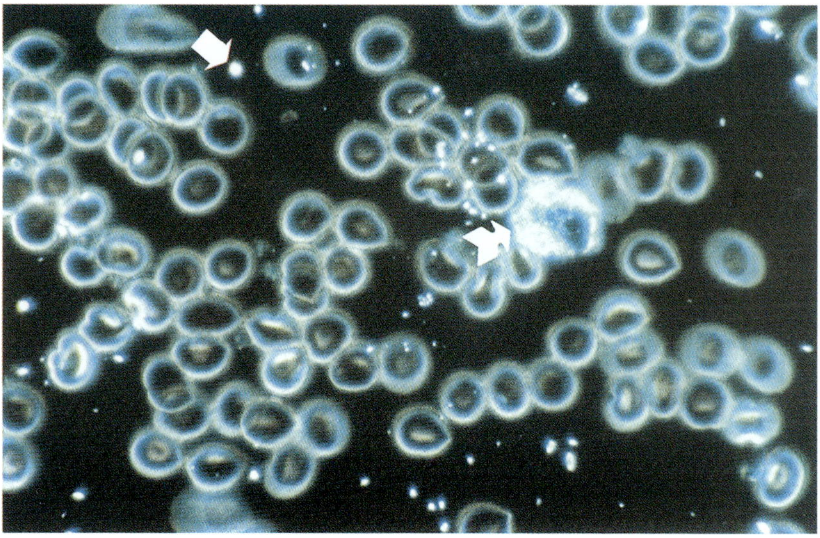

Aufnahme von: 9/1988 – Photo taken: 9/1988

Bewertung: ➽ Granulozyt von parasitären Symprotiten befallen (Kern und Plasma) – Abwehrschwäche; Erythrozyten endobiontisch belastet, zitronenförmige E. – Leberbelastung; im Blutplasma sporoide Symprotiten ➡.

Evaluation: ➽ Granulocyte infested with parasitic symprotits (nucleus and plasma) – defence weakness; erythrocytes endobiontically infested, lemon-shaped erythrocytes – liver stress; ➡ sporoid symprotits in the blood plasma.

Patientin: R., geb. 1920
Diagnose: Gallenstau, OP Zyste am Leberlappen links

Patient (female): R., born 1920
Diagnosis: Gall congestion, operation of cyst on the left lobe of the liver

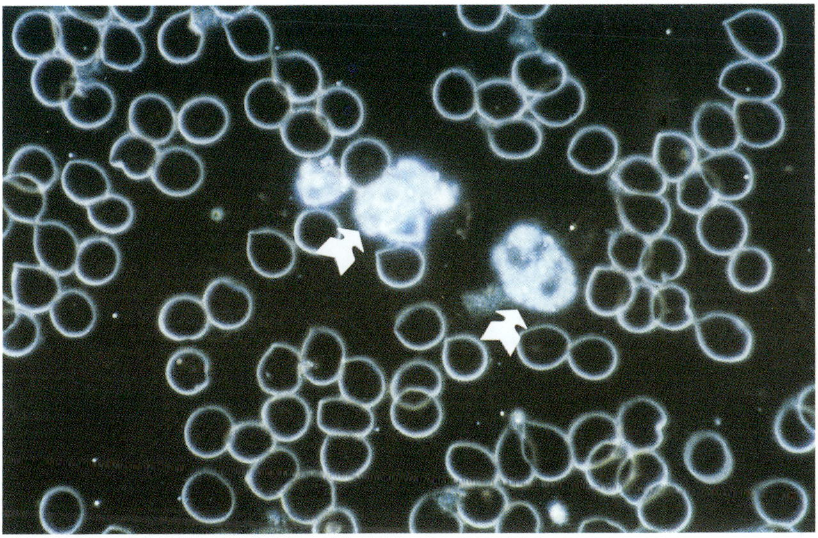

Aufnahme von: 5/1989 – Photo taken: 5/1989

Bewertung: ➽ Mehrere von parasitären Symprotiten befallene Granulozyten – zelluläre Abwehr geschwächt; zitronenförmige Erythrozyten – Leberbelastung.

Evaluation: ➽ Several granulocytes infested with parasitic symprotits – cellular defence weakened; lemon-shaped erythrocytes – liver stress.

Patientin: K., geb. 1969
Diagnose: Chronische Cystitis, chronische Sinusitis (Fehldiagnose MS)

Patient (female): K., born 1969
Diagnosis: Chronic cystitis, chronic sinusitis (false diagnosis of multiple sclerosis)

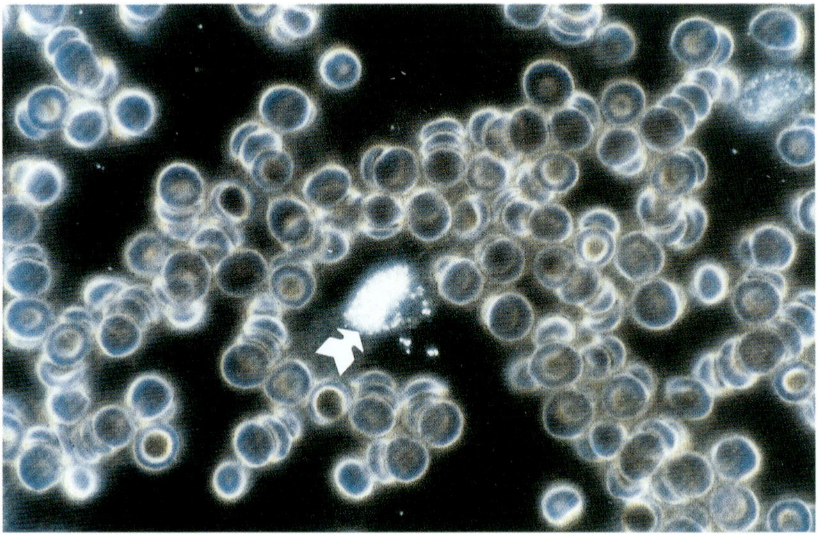

Aufnahme von: 10/1990 – Photo taken: 10/1990

Bewertung: ➽ Mit parasitären Symprotiten befallener, in Auflösung begriffener Granulozyt – zelluläre Abwehr geschwächt; Endobiose der Erythrozyten.

Evaluation: ➽ Granulocyte, infested with parasitic symprotits, in state of degradation – weakened cellular defence; endobiosis of the erythrocytes.

Patientin: A., geb. 1955
Diagnose: Allergische Diathese

Patient (female): A., born 1955
Diagnosis: Allergical diathesis

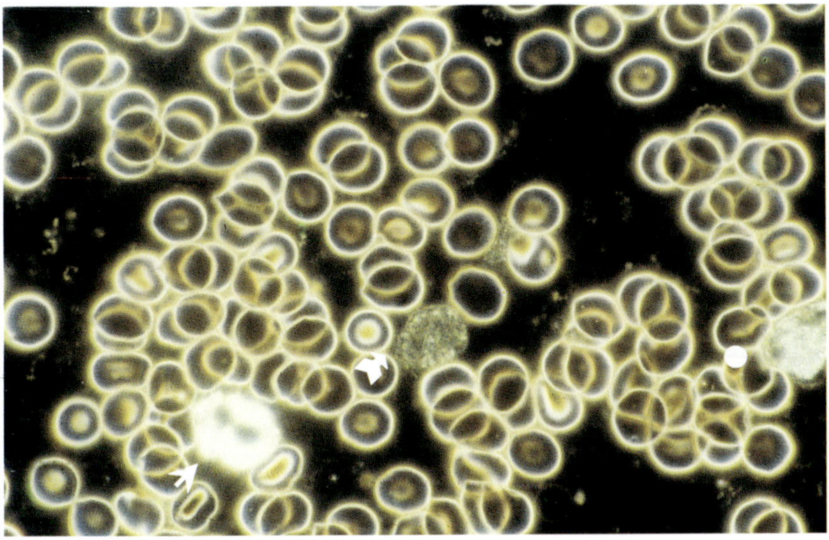

Aufnahme von: 3/1995 – Photo taken: 3/1995

Bewertung: 3 Leukozyten, ↗ in der linken unteren Bildhälfte eosinophiler Granulozyt; ⇗ in der Bildmitte kleiner Monozyt;
● rechts neutrophiler Granulozyt.

Evaluation: 3 leucocytes, ↗ on the left eosinophile granulocyte;
⇗ in the centre little monocyte;
● on the right neutrophile granulocyte.

Patient:	K., geb. 1938
Diagnose:	Thrombophlebitis, Ulcus cruris an beiden Beinen, Skoliose, Gonarthrose

Patient:	K., born 1938
Diagnosis:	Thrombophlebitis, varicose ulcer on both legs, scoliosis, gonarthrosis

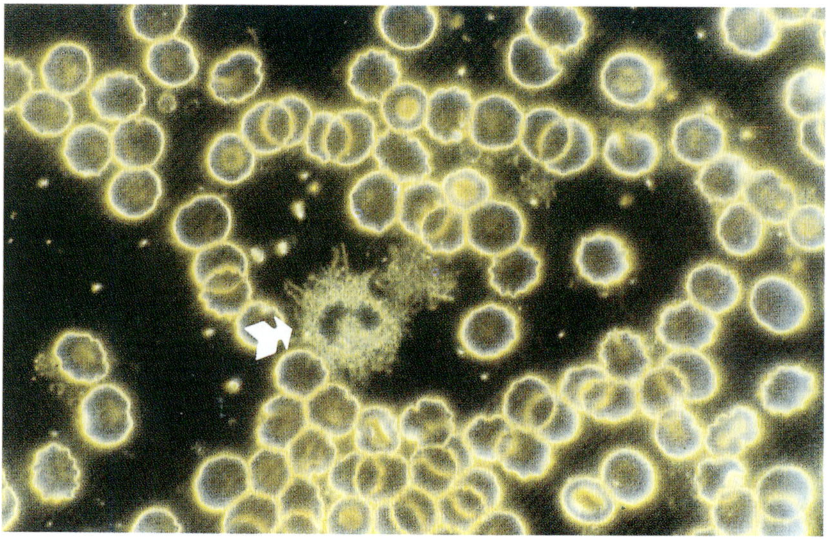

Aufnahme von: 7/1992 – Photo taken: 7/1992

Bewertung: ➽ Zerfallender Leukozyt mit Chondrit-Dendroiden, Leukozytenmaterial vom Endobionten fast völlig verbraucht – zelluläre Abwehr kommt zum Erliegen (nach 4 Stunden).

Evaluation: ➽ Leucocyte in state of degradation with chondrit-dendroids, leucocytic material nearly completely used up by the endobiont – cellular defence is coming to a standstill (after four hours).

Patientin: R., geb. 1945
Diagnose: Osteomyelosklerose

Patient (female): R., born 1945
Diagnosis: Osteomyelosclerosis

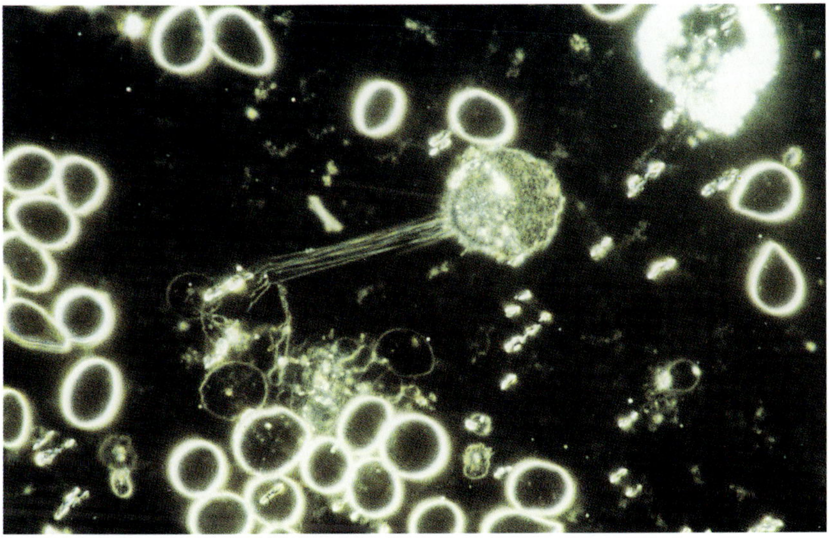

Aufnahme von: 2/1999 – Photo taken: 2/1999

Bewertung: Nicht ausgereifter Leukozyt mit langen Pseudopodien (= Chrondrit-dendroide) – befallener Leukozyt versucht die parasitären Formen des Endobionten zu entsorgen (nach 2 Stunden).

Evaluation: Leucocyte with pseudopodias (= chrondrit-dendroids) – infested leucocyte tries to "remove the waste" of the parasitic forms of the endobiont (after two hours).

Patientin: E., geb. 1921
Diagnose: Urathische Diathese

Patient (female): E., born 1921
Diagnosis: Urathic diathesis

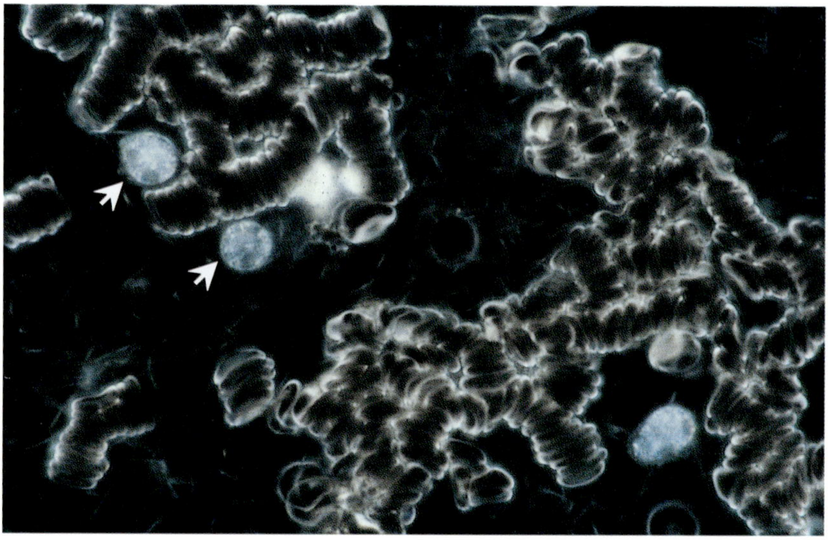

Aufnahme von: 2/1989 – Photo taken: 2/1989

Bewertung: ➚ Kleine unbewegliche kreisrunde neutrophile Granulozyten – zelluläre Abwehr blockiert.

Evaluation: ➚ Little immovable round granulocytes – blocked cellular defence.

Patientin: P., geb. 1987
Diagnose: Neurodermitis, Alopecie

Patient (female): P., born 1987
Diagnosis: Neurodermitis, alopecia

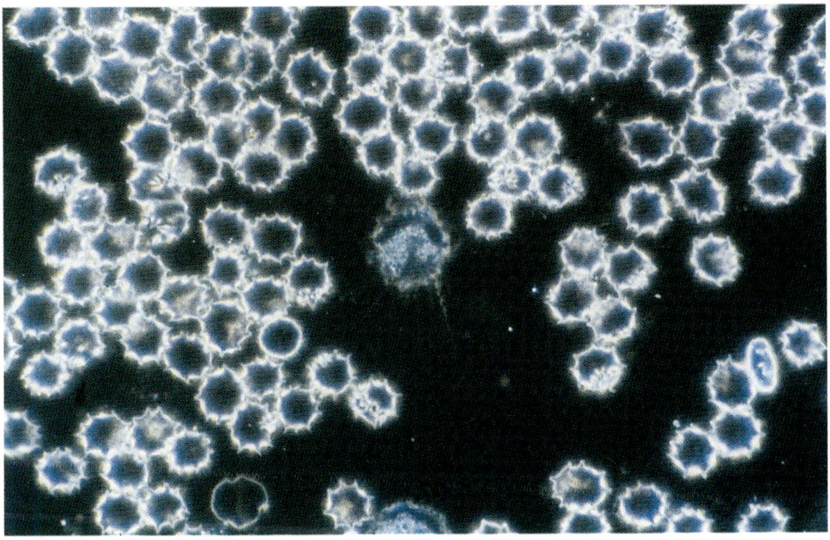

Aufnahme von: 10/1990 – Photo taken: 10/1990

Bewertung: In der Mitte Granulozyt mit Pseudopodien (= Chondrit-Dendroid des Endobionten) – „Entsorgung" der parasitären Formen des Endobionten; Erythrozyten endobiontisch belastet (12 h nach Blutentnahme).

Evaluation: In the centre granulocyte with pseudopodias (= chondrit-dendroid of the endobiont) – „removal of waste" of the parasitic forms of the endobiont; erythrocytes endobiontically burdened (12 hours after taking a blood sample).

Patient:	P., geb. 1926
Diagnose:	Polyglobulie, Cholelithiasis, Nephritis, Cystitis

Patient:	P., born 1926
Diagnosis:	Polyglobulia, cholelithiasis, nephritis, cystitis

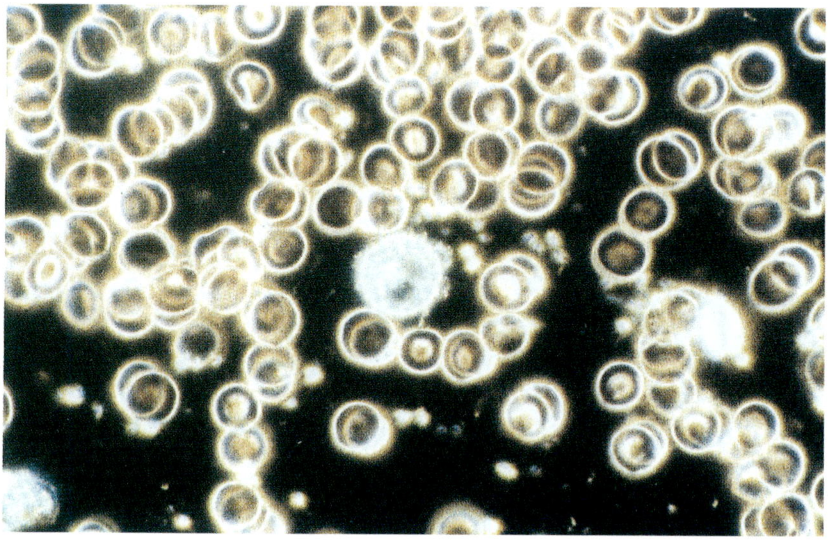

Aufnahme von: 12/1992 – Photo taken: 12/1992

Bewertung: Skierotisierter Leukozyt in der Bildmitte – Abwehr geschwächt; Endobiose der Erythrozyten (1 h nach Blutentnahme).

Evaluation: Sclerosed leucocyte in the centre of the picture – weakened defence; endobiosis of the erythrocytes (one hour after taking a blood sample).

Patient: F., geb. 1966
Diagnose: Apoplex, Durchblutungsstörungen

Patient: F., born 1966
Diagnosis: Apoplexia, disturbances of blood supply

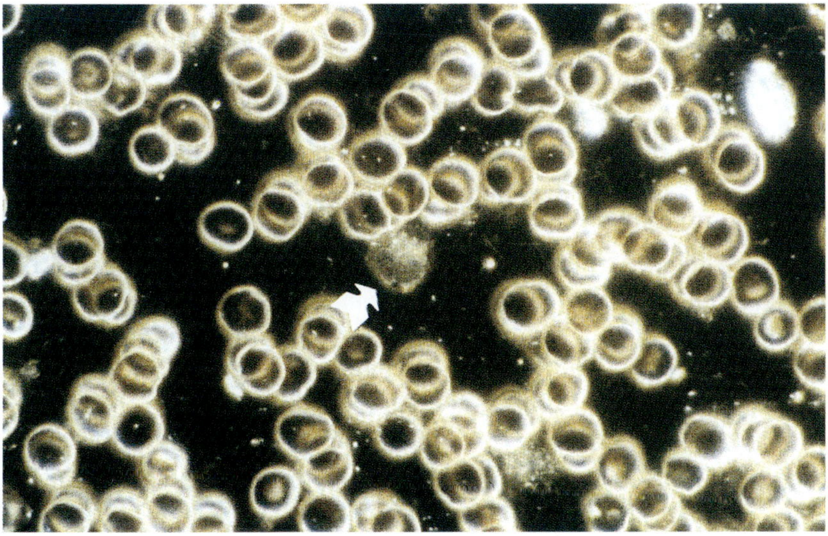

Aufnahme von: 9/1992 – Photo taken: 9/1992

Bewertung: ➽ In der Bildmitte Monozyt, der von parasitären Symprotiten befallen ist – zelluläre Abwehr beeinträchtigt.

Evaluation: ➽ In the centre of the picture monocyte that is infested with parasitic symprotits – impaired cellular defence.

Patient: M., geb. 1948
Diagnose: Durchblutungsstörungen, Immunschwäche

Patient: M., born 1948
Diagnosis: Disturbances of blood supply, immunological weakness

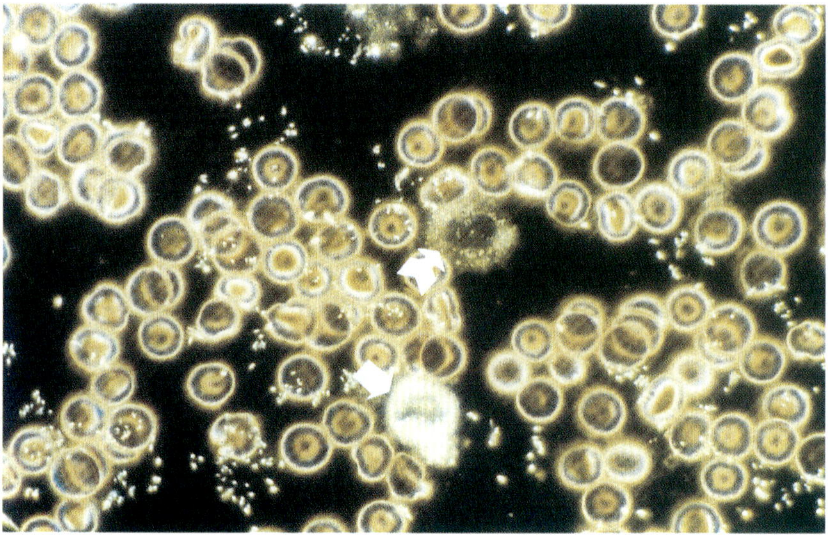

Aufnahme von: 1/1993 – Photo taken: 1/1993

Bewertung: ➽ In Bildmitte zerfallender Leukozyt, dessen Kernmaterial vom Endobionten fast vollständig verbraucht wurde; ➡ am unteren Bildrand mit parasitären Symprotiten befallener Leukozyt – geschwächte zelluläre Abwehr; Endobiose der Erythrozyten (1 h nach Blutentnahme).

Evaluation: ➽ In the centre of the picture leucocyte in state of degradation, the nucleus material of which has been nearly completely used up; ➡ on the lower edge of the picture leucocyte infested with parasitic symprotits – weakened cellular defence; endobiosis of the erythrocytes (one hour after taking a blood sample).

Patient: P., geb. 1908
Diagnose: Blasen-Ca, Durchblutungsstörungen in beiden Beinen, Angina pectoris, Gastritis, Colitis ulcerosa

Patient: P., born 1908
Diagnosis: Carcinoma of the bladder, disturbances of blood supply in both legs, angina pectoris, gastritis, ulcerous colitis

Aufnahme 1 – Photo 1

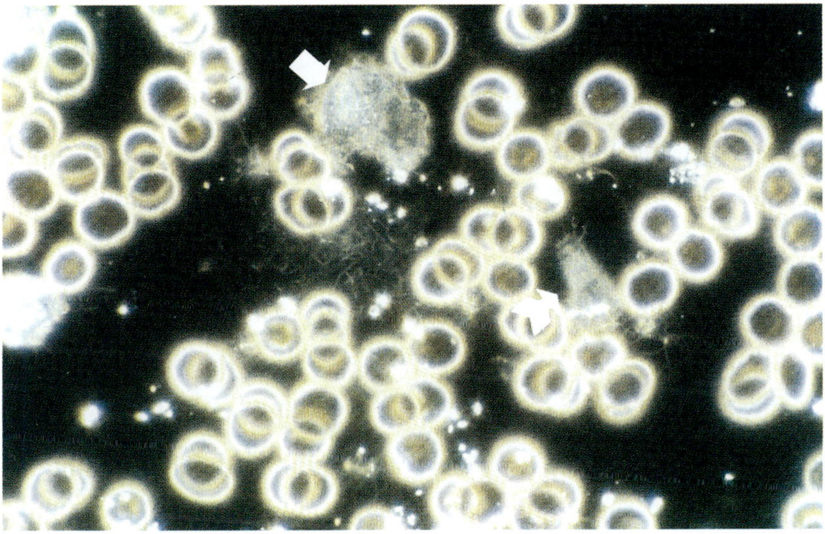

Aufnahme von: 1/1993 – Photo taken: 1/1993

Bewertung: Endobiontisch befallene Leukozyten, ➽ ovaler Lymphozyt in rechter Bildhälfte mit Chondrit-Dendroiden, am oberem Bildrand 2 zusammengeballte entartete Monozyten ➡ die von sporoiden Symprotiten befallen sind – schwache zelluläre Abwehr, schwerstes Krankheitsbild (1 h nach Blutentnahme).

Evaluation: Endobiontically infested leucocytes, in the right half of the picture ➽ oval lymphocyte with chondrit-dendroids, on the upper edge of the picture 2 massed, degenerated monocytes ➡ that are infested with sporoid symprotits - weak cellular defence, extremely severe pathological picture (one hour after taking a blood sample).

Patient: P., geb. 1908
Diagnose: Blasen-Ca, Durchblutungsstörungen in beiden Beinen, Angina pectoris, Gastritis, Colitis ulcerosa

Patient: P., born 1908
Diagnosis: Carcinoma of the bladder, disturbances of blood supply in both legs, angina pectoris, gastritis, ulcerous colitis

Aufnahme 2 – Photo 2

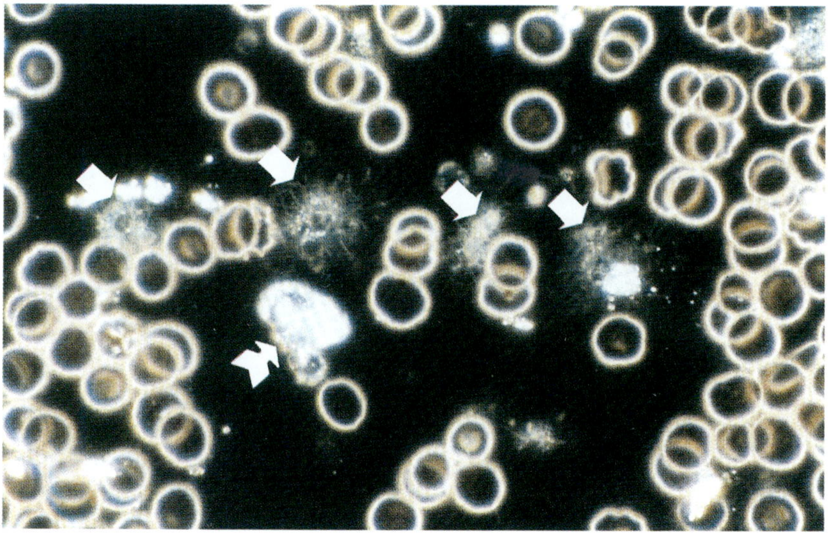

Aufnahme von: 1/1993 – Photo taken: 1/1993

Bewertung: ➽ Endobiontisch befallener Granulozyt, 4 in Chondrit-Dendroide zerfallene Lymphozyten ➡ – zelluläre Abwehr blockiert (1 h nach Blutentnahme).

Evaluation: ➽ Endobiontically infested granulocyte, 4 lymphocytes degrading into chondrit-dendroids ➡ – blocked cellular defence (one hour after taking a blood sample).

Patient:	P., geb. 1908
Diagnose:	Blasen-Ca, Durchblutungsstörungen in beiden Beinen, Angina pectoris, Gastritis, Colitis ulcerosa

Patient:	P., born 1908
Diagnosis:	Carcinoma of the bladder, disturbances of blood supply in both legs, angina pectoris, gastritis, ulcerous colitis

Aufnahme 3 – Photo 3

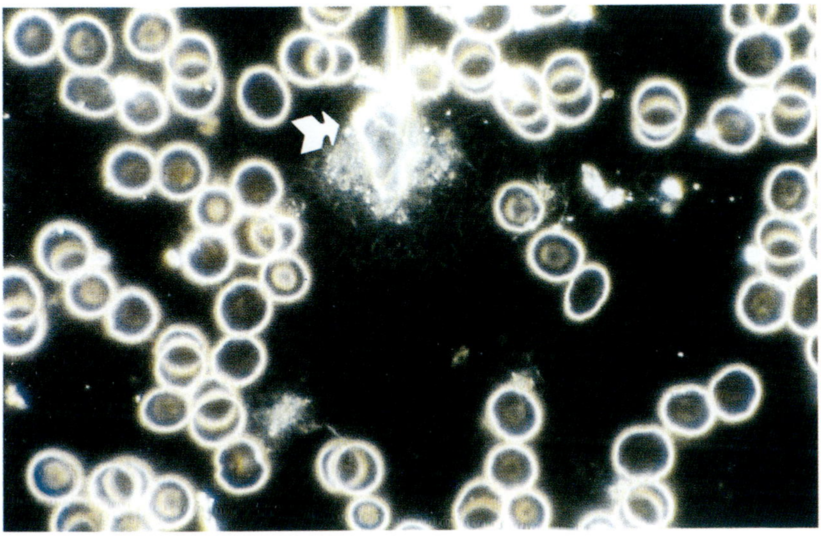

Aufnahme von: 1/1993 – Photo taken: 1/1993

Bewertung: ➽ Obere Bildhälfte mit Pseudokristall aus Oberbauch, der von 2 Leukozyten attackiert wurde, die in Chondrit-Dendroide zerfallen sind – schlechte Abwehrlage (1 h nach Blutentnahme).

Evaluation: ➽ Upper half of picture with pseudocrystals from upper abdomen, which was attacked by two leucocytes that have disintegrated into chondrit-dendroids – bad defence condition (1 hour after the taking of a blood sample).

Patientin:	Sch., geb. 1914
Diagnose:	Leukämie, Osteomyelitis

Patient (female):	Sch., born 1914
Diagnosis:	Leucemia, osteomyelitis

Aufnahme 2 – Photo 2

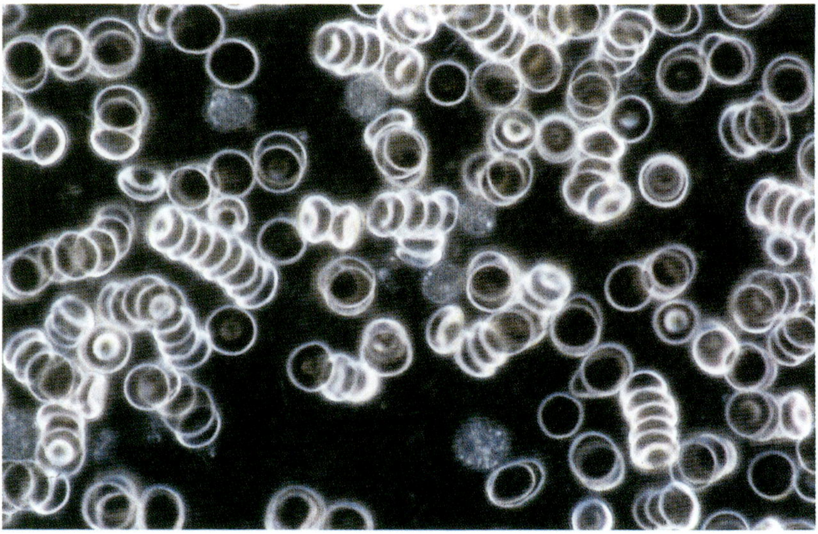

Aufnahme von: 10/1989 – Photo taken: 10/1989

Bewertung: Nach 3 Monaten verminderte Agglutination der Erythrozyten.

Evaluation: After 3 months reduced agglutination of the erythrocytes.

Patientin: Sch., geb. 1914
Diagnose: Leukämie, Osteomyelitis

Patient (female): Sch., born 1914
Diagnosis: Leucemia, osteomyelitis

Aufnahme 3 – Photo 3

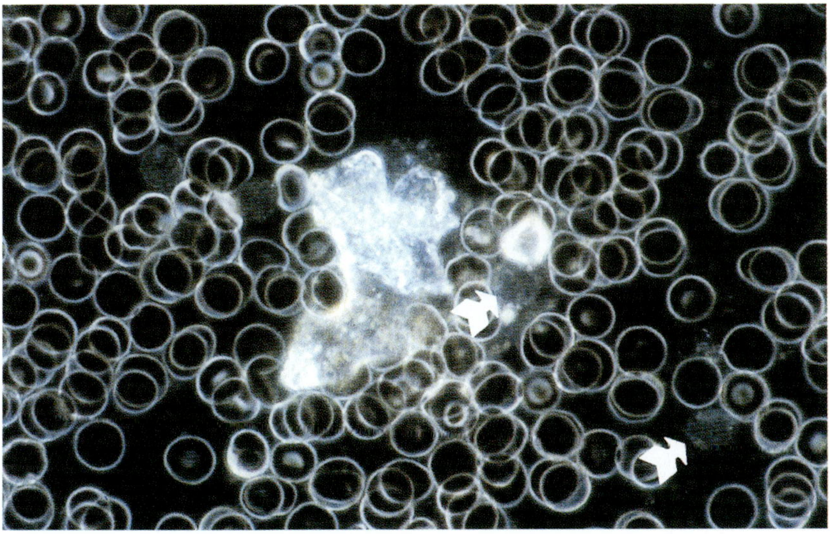

Aufnahme von: 10/1989 – Photo taken: 10/1989

Bewertung: Sklerotisches Gebilde in der Mitte, rechts davon 2 Lymphozyten ➽.

Evaluation: In the centre sclerotic formation, next to the right 2 lymphocytes ➽.

Patientin: Th., geb. 1914
Diagnose: 1988 Apoplex, Diabetes mellitus, chronische Sinusitis

Patient (female): Th., born 1914
Diagnosis: 1988 apoplexia, alimentary diabetes, chronic sinusitis

Aufnahme 1 – Photo 1

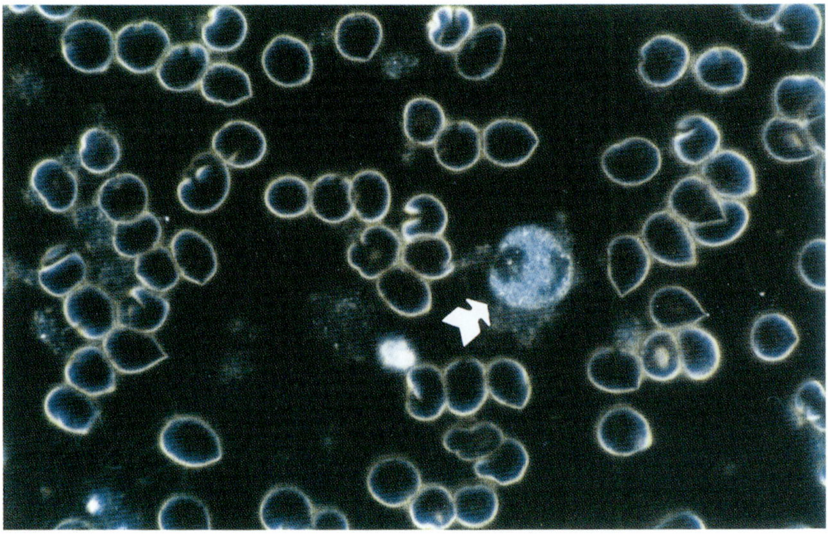

Aufnahme von: 5/1989 – Photo taken: 5/1989

Bewertung: ➽ Leukozyt, der von parasitären Symprotiten befallen ist – zelluläre Abwehr geschwächt; zitronenförmige Erythrozyten – Leberbelastung.

Evaluation: ➽ Leucocyte infested with parasitic symprotits – weakened cellular defence; lemon-shaped erythrocytes – liver stress.

Patientin:	Th., geb. 1914
Diagnose:	1988 Apoplex, Diabetes mellitus, chronische Sinusitis

Patient (female):	Th., born 1914
Diagnosis:	1988 apoplexia, alimentary diabetes, chronic sinusitis

Aufnahme 2 – Photo 2

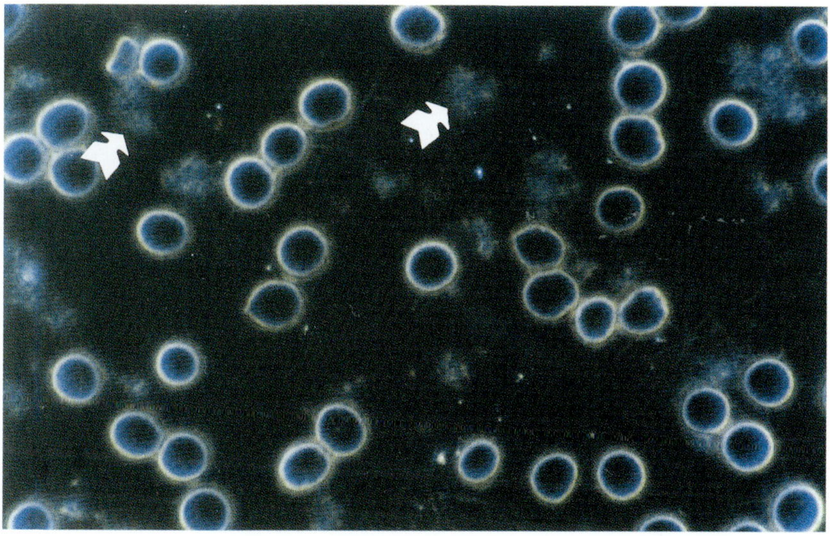

Aufnahme von: 5/1989 – Photo taken: 5/1989

Bewertung: ➽ Zusammengeballte Thrombozyten – Stauungen; stark leuchtende Erythrozytenmembranen.

Evaluation: ➽ Massed thrombocytes – congestions; brightly shining membranes of the erythrocytes.

Patientin:	Th., geb. 1914
Diagnose:	1988 Apoplex, Diabetes mellitus, chronische Sinusitis

Patient (female):	Th., born 1914
Diagnosis:	1988 apoplexia, alimentary diabetes, chronic sinusitis

Aufnahme 3 – Photo 3

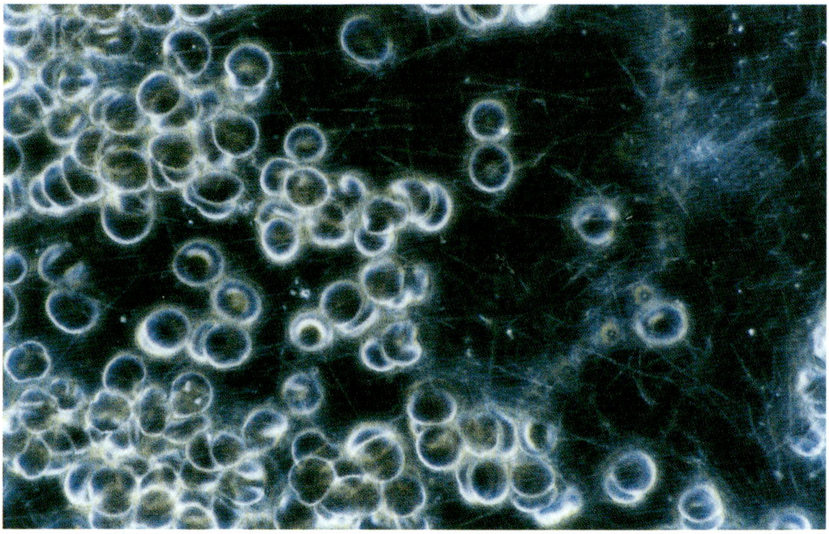

Aufnahme von: 5/1989 – Photo taken: 5/1989

Bewertung:	Filitbildung – Stauungen,- Agglutination der Erythrozyten – endobiontische Belastung.
Evaluation:	Filit formation – congestions; agglutination of the erythrocytes – endobiontic burden.

Beobachtung eines Blutbildes bis zum Zerfall

Patientin: Sch., geb. 1955
Diagnose: Durchblutungsstörungen in den Extremitäten, Darmmykose

Patient (female): Sch., born 1955
Diagnosis: Disturbances of blood supply in the extremities, intestine mycosis

Aufnahme 1 – Photo 1

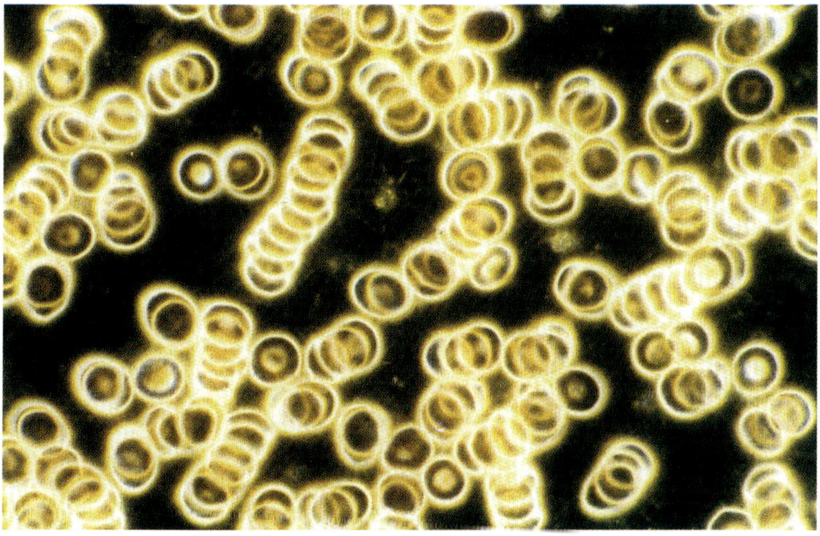

Aufnahme von: 12/1993 – Photo taken: 12/1993

Bewertung: Agglutination der Erythrozyten in Form von Geldrollen – Stauungen.

Evaluation: Agglutination of the erythrocytes in formations of coin rolls – congestion.

Patientin: Sch., geb. 1955
Diagnose: Durchblutungsstörungen in den Extremitäten, Darmmykose

Patient (female): Sch., born 1955
Diagnosis: Disturbances of blood supply in the extremities, intestine mycosis

Aufnahme 2 – Photo 2

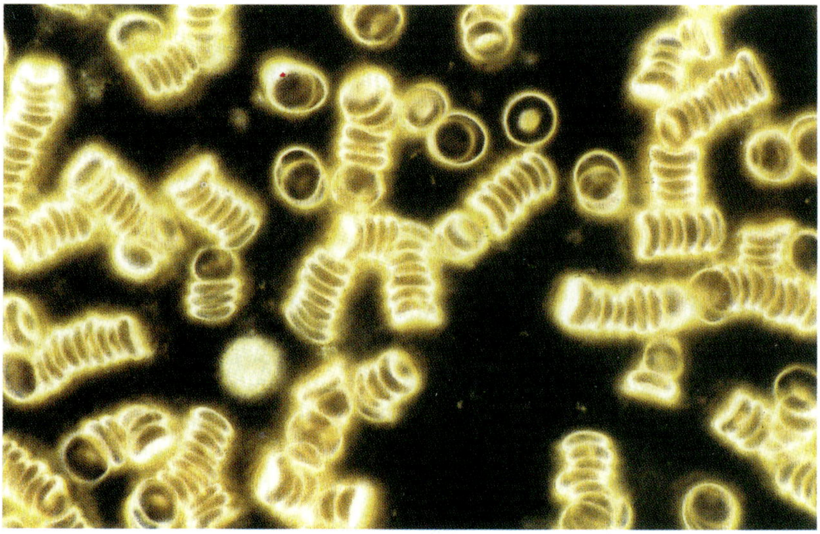

Aufnahme von: 12/1993 – Photo taken: 12/1993

Bewertung: Nach zwei Stunden: Agglutination der Erythrozyten verstärkt sich – chronisches Geschehen.

Evaluation: After two hours: Agglutination of the erythrocytes is increasing – chronic process.

Patientin: Sch., geb. 1955
Diagnose: Durchblutungsstörungen in den Extremitäten, Darmmykose

Patient (female): Sch., born 1955
Diagnosis: Disturbances of blood supply in the extremities, intestine mycosis

Aufnahme 3 – Photo 3

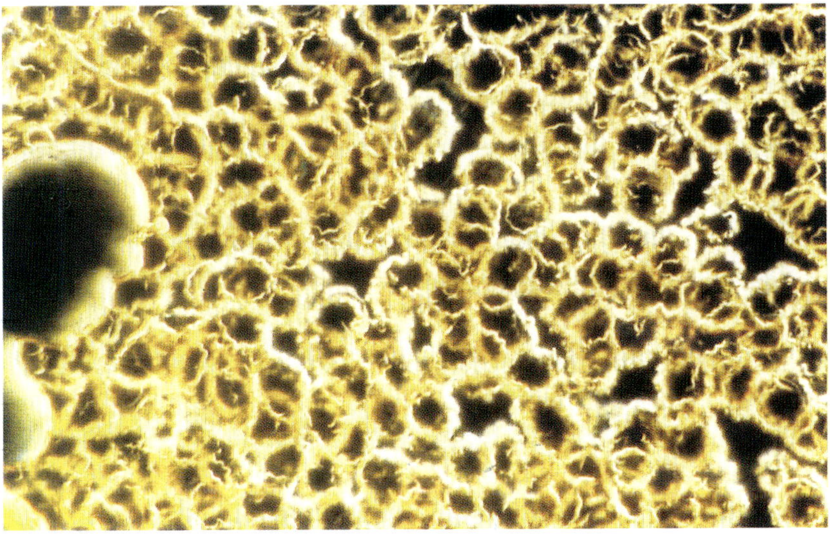

Aufnahme von: 12/1993 – Photo taken: 12/1993

Bewertung: Zerfall des Blutbildes nach 18 Stunden – chronische Erkrankung.

Evaluation: Disintegration of the blood picture after 18 hours – chronic disease.